CHILDREN'S ISSUES, LAWS AND PROGRAMS

SOLVING CHILDHOOD OBESITY

CHILDREN'S ISSUES, LAWS AND PROGRAMS

Additional books in this series can be found on Nova's website
under the Series tab.

Additional E-books in this series can be found on Nova's website
under the E-books tab.

NUTRITION AND DIET RESEARCH PROGRESS

Additional books in this series can be found on Nova's website
under the Series tab.

Additional E-books in this series can be found on Nova's website
under the E-books tab.

CHILDREN'S ISSUES, LAWS AND PROGRAMS

SOLVING CHILDHOOD OBESITY

SARAH J. MAIER
AND
NATALIE E. BRUNNER
EDITORS

Nova Science Publishers, Inc.
New York

For permission to use material from this book please contact us:
Telephone 631-231-7269; Fax 631-231-8175
Web Site: http://www.novapublishers.com

Library of Congress Cataloging-in-Publication Data

Solving childhood obesity / [edited by] Sarah J. Maier and Natalie E.Brunner.
p. cm.
Includes index.
ISBN 978-1-61209-964-4 (hardcover)
1. Obesity in children--United States--Prevention. 2. Overweight children--United States. I. Maier, Sarah J. II. Brunner, Natalie E.
RJ399.C6S655 2011
618.92'398--dc22

2011005843

Published by Nova Science Publishers, Inc. † New York

CONTENTS

PREFACE

The childhood obesity epidemic in America is a national health crisis. One in every three children ages 2-19 is overweight or obese. The life-threatening consequences of this epidemic create a compelling and critical call for action that cannot be ignored. Obesity is estimated to cause 112,000 deaths per year in the United States, and one third of all children born in the year 2000 are expected to develop diabetes during their lifetime. The current generation may even be on track to have a shorter lifespan than their parents. This new book focuses on the research and scientific information on the causes and consequences of childhood obesity which form the platform on which to build our national policies and partner with the private sector to end the childhood obesity epidemic.

Chapter 1- The childhood obesity epidemic in America is a national health crisis One in every three children (31.7%) ages 2-19 is overweight or obese.[1] The life-threatening consequences of this epidemic create a compelling and critical call for action that cannot be ignored Obesity is estimated to cause 112,000 deaths per year in the United States,[2] and one third of all children born in the year 2000 are expected to develop diabetes during their lifetime.[3] The current generation may even be on track to have a shorter lifespan than their parents.[4]

Chapter 2- In children and adolescents, obesity is defined as being at or above the 95th percentile of the age- and sex-specific body mass index (BMI); overweight is defined as being between the 85th and 94th percentiles, based on growth charts developed by the Centers for Disease Control and Prevention. The National Health and Nutrition Examination Survey has gathered data showing that, over the past three decades, obesity rates have tripled among children and adolescents. Today, about 32% of U.S. children and adolescents between the ages of 2 and 19 are overweight, and more than half of those children are considered obese.

Chapter 3- Our nation stands at a crossroads. Today's epidemic of overweight and obesity threatens the historic progress we have made in increasing American's quality and years of healthy life. Two-third of adults[1] and nearly one in three children are overweight or obese.[2] In addition, many racial and ethnic groups and geographic regions of the United States are disproportionately affected.[3] The sobering impact of these numbers is reflected in the nation's concurrent epidemics of diabetes, heart disease, and other chronic diseases. If we do not reverse these trends, researchers warn that many of our children—our most precious resource—will be seriously afflicted in early adulthood with medical conditions such as diabetes and heart disease. This future is unacceptable. The author asks you to join in combating this crisis.

Chapter 4- Childhood obesity continues to be a leading public health concern that disproportionately affects low-income and minority children [1]. Children who are obese in their preschool years are more likely to be obese in adolescence and adulthood [2] and to develop diabetes, hypertension, hyperlipidemia, asthma, and sleep apnea [3]. One of the *Healthy People 2010* objectives (19-3) is to reduce to 5% the proportion of children and adolescents who are obese [4]. CD C's Pediatric Nutrition Surveillance System (PedNSS) is the only source of nationally compiled obesity surveillance data obtained at the state and local level for low-income, preschool-aged children participating in federally funded health and nutrition programs. To describe progress in reducing childhood obesity, CDC examined trends and current prevalence in obesity using PedNSS data submitted by participating states, territories, and Indian tribal organizations during 1998–2008. The findings indicated that obesity prevalence among low-income, preschool-aged children increased steadily from 12.4% in 1998 to 14.5% in 2003, but subsequently remained essentially the same, with a 14.6% prevalence in 2008. Reducing childhood obesity will require effective prevention strategies that focus on environments and policies promoting physical activity and a healthy diet for families, child care centers, and communities.

Chapter 5- Although there is a long history of public concern over the impact of mass media on children's psychosocial development (Center on Media and Child Health 2005; Lowery and DeFleur 1995), it is only in the past two decades that researchers have begun to uncover the link between media use and the physical health of youths. Data from large-scale national surveys conducted during the 1980s and 1990s reveal a correlation between the prevalence of overweight and the number of hours youths spend watching TV (Andersen et al. 1998; Dietz and Gortmaker 1985). More importantly, subsequent longitudinal studies (Gortmaker et al. 1996) and field experiments (Robinson1999) have indicated a potential causal connection between obesity/overweight and heavy TV use.

In: Solving Childhood Obesity
Editors: Sarah J. Maier and Natalie E. Brunner

ISBN: 978-1-61209-964-4

Chapter 1

SOLVING THE PROBLEM OF CHILDHOOD OBESITY WITHIN A GENERATION

White House Task Force on Childhood Obesity, Report to the President

THE CHALLENGE WE FACE

The childhood obesity epidemic in America is a national health crisis One in every three children (31.7%) ages 2-19 is overweight or obese.[1] The life-threatening consequences of this epidemic create a compelling and critical call for action that cannot be ignored Obesity is estimated to cause 112,000 deaths per year in the United States,[2] and one third of all children born in the year 2000 are expected to develop diabetes during their lifetime.[3] The current generation may even be on track to have a shorter lifespan than their parents.[4]

Along with the effects on our children's health, childhood obesity imposes substantial economic costs. Each year, obese adults incur an estimated $1,429 more in medical expenses than their normal-weight peers.[5] Overall, medical spending on adults that was attributed to obesity topped approximately $40 billion in 1998, and by 2008, increased to an estimated $147 billion.[6] Excess weight is also costly during childhood, estimated at $3 billion per year in direct medical costs. [7]

Childhood obesity also creates potential implications for military readiness. More than one quarter of all Americans ages 17-24 are unqualified for military service because they are too heavy.[8] As one military leader noted recently, "We have an obesity crisis in the country. There's no question about it. These are the same young people we depend on to serve in times of need and ultimately protect this nation." [9]

While these statistics are striking, there is much reason to be hopeful. There is considerable knowledge about the risk factors associated with childhood obesity. Research and scientific information on the causes and consequences of childhood obesity form the platform on which to build our national policies and partner with the private sector to end the childhood obesity epidemic. Effective policies and tools to guide healthy eating and active living are within our grasp. This report will focus and expand on what we can do together to:

1. create a healthy start on life for our children, from pregnancy through early childhood;
2. empower parents and caregivers to make healthy choices for their families;
3. serve healthier food in schools;
4. ensure access to healthy, affordable food; and
5. increase opportunities for physical activity.

What is Obesity?

Obesity is defined as excess body fat. Because body fat is difficult to measure directly, obesity is often measured by body mass index (BMI), a common scientific way to screen for whether a person is underweight, normal weight, overweight, or obese. BMI adjusts weight for height,[10] and while it is not a perfect indicator of obesity,[11] it is a valuable tool for public health.

Adults with a BMI between 25.0 and 29.9 are considered overweight, those with a BMI of 30 or more are considered obese, and those with a BMI of 40 or more are considered extremely obese.[12] For children and adolescents, these BMI categories are further divided by sex and age because of the changes that occur during growth and development. Growth charts from the Centers for Disease Control and Prevention (CDC) are used to calculate children's BMI. Children and adolescents with a BMI between the 85th and 94th percentiles are generally considered overweight, and those with a BMI at or above the sex-and age-specific 95th percentile of population on this growth chart are typically considered obese.

Determining what is a healthy weight for children is challenging, even with precise measures. BMI is often used as a screening tool, since a BMI in the overweight or obese range often, but not always, indicates that a child is at increased risk for health problems. A clinical assessment and other indicators must also be considered when evaluating a child's overall health and development.[13]

Who Does Obesity Impact? Prevalence and Trends

By gaining a deeper understanding of individuals who are impacted by obesity, we can better shape policies to combat it. Since 1980, obesity has become dramatically more common among Americans of all ages. Prevalence estimates of obesity in the U. S. are derived from the National Health and Nutrition Examination Survey (NHANES), conducted by the National Center for Health Statistics of the CDC. Between the survey periods 1976–80 and 2007–08, obesity has more than doubled among adults (rising from 15% to 34%), and more than tripled among children and adolescents (rising from 5% to 17%).[14]

The rapid increase in childhood obesity in the 1980s and 1990s has slowed, with no significant increase in recent years.[15] However, among boys ages 6–19, very high BMI (at or above the 97th percentile) became more common between 1999–2000 and 2007–08; about 15% of boys in this age group are in this category. [16]

Race/Ethnic Disparities

Childhood obesity is more common among certain racial and ethnic groups than others Obesity rates are highest among non-Hispanic black girls and Hispanic boys. Obesity is particularly common among American Indian/Native Alaskan children. A study of four year-olds found that obesity was more than two times more common among American Indian/Native Alaskan children (31%) than among white (16%) or Asian (13%) children. This rate was higher than any other racial or ethnic group studied. [17]

Socioeconomic Disparities

Among adults, obesity rates are sometimes associated with lower incomes, particularly among women. Women with higher incomes tend to have lower BMI, and the opposite is true, those with higher BMI have lower incomes.[18] A study in the early 2000s found that about 38% of non-Hispanic white women who qualified for the Supplemental Nutrition Assistance Program (known then as food stamps), were obese, and about 26% of those above 350% of the poverty line were obese. [19] Also, a recent study of American adults found lower rates of obesity among individuals with more education. Specifically, the study found that nearly 35% of adults with less than a high school degree were obese, compared to 21% of those with a bachelor's degree or higher. [20]

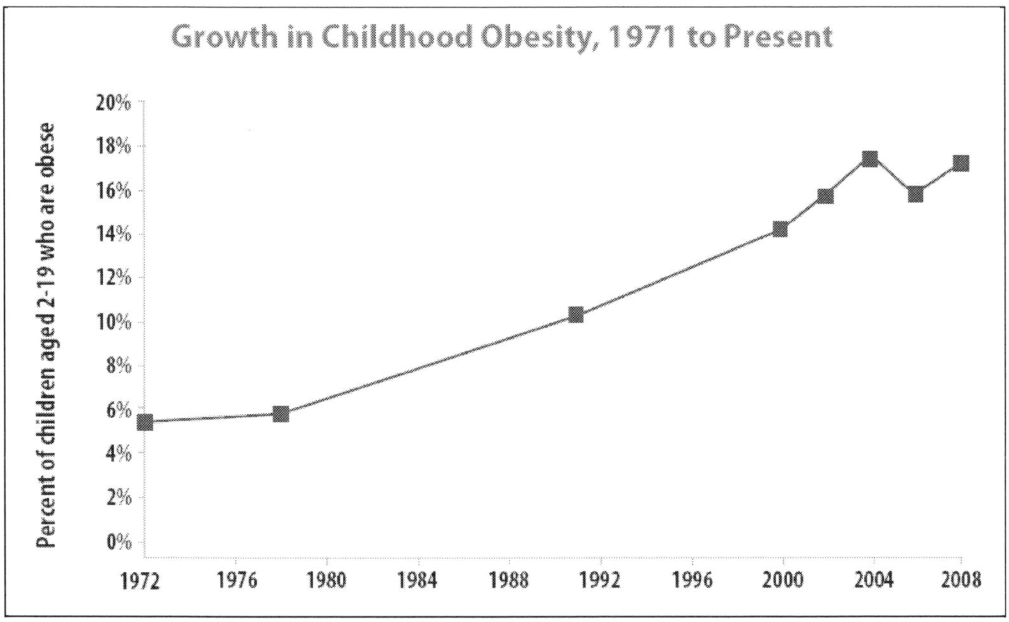

Source: CDC, National Center for Health Statistics, National Health and Nutrition Examination Surveys.

Note: Obesity is defined as BMI ≥ gender- and weight-specific 95th percentile from the 2000 CDC Growth Charts.

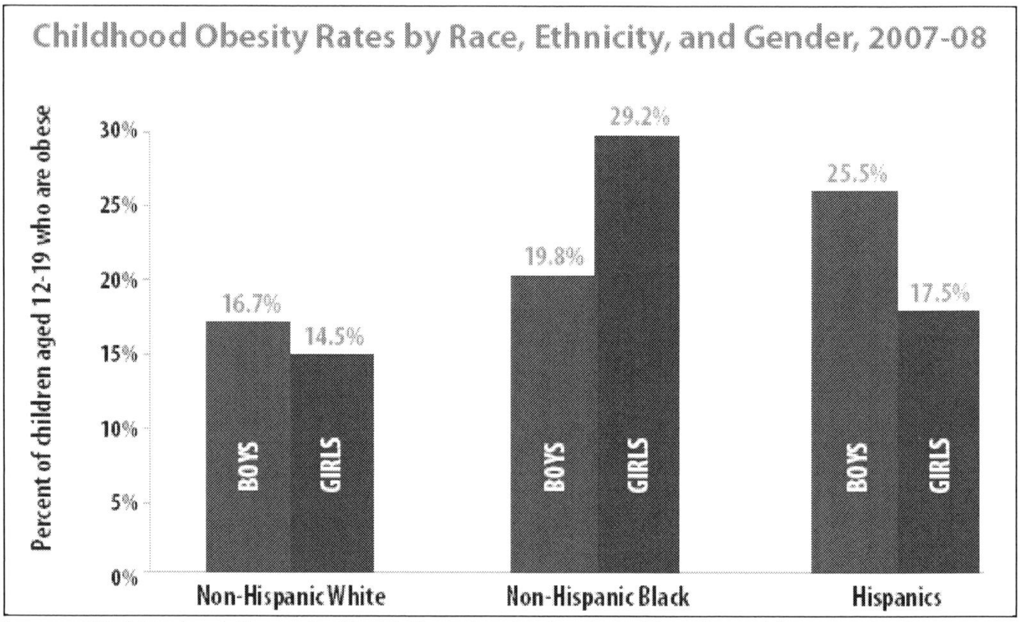

Source: CDC, National Center for Health Statistics, National Health and Nutrition Examination Survey;
Note: Obesity is defined as BMI ≥ gender- and weight-specific 95th percentile from the 2000 CDC Growth Charts.

The relationship between income and obesity in children is less consistent than among adult women,[21] and sometimes even points in the opposite direction. Another study from the early 2000s found that only among white girls were higher incomes associated with lower BMI. Among African-American girls, the prevalence of obesity actually increased with higher socioeconomic status, suggesting that efforts to reduce ethnic disparities in obesity must target factors other than income and education, such as environmental, social, and cultural factors. [22]

Regional Disparities

Across the country, the prevalence of obesity has been found to be highest in southeast states such as Alabama, Mississippi, South Carolina, Tennessee, and West Virginia, as well as in Oklahoma. It is lowest in Colorado.[23] Another study showed obesity was most common among adults in the Midwest and the South, as well as among adults who did not live in metropolitan areas.[24]

How Does Obesity Impact Our Health?

Obese adults have an increased risk for many diseases, including type 2 diabetes, heart disease, some forms of arthritis, and several cancers.[25] Overweight and obese children are more likely to become obese adults.[26] Specifically, one study found that obese 6-8 year-olds were approximately ten times more likely to become obese adults than those with lower BMIs.[27] The association may be stronger for obese adolescents than younger children.[28] Obese children are also more likely to have increased risk of heart disease.[29] One study found that approximately 70% of obese children had high levels (greater than 90th percentile) of at least one key risk factor for heart disease, and approximately 30% had high levels of at least two risk factors.[30] There is evidence that heart disease develops in early childhood and is exacerbated by obesity,[31] and people as young as 21 have been found to display early physical signs of heart disease due to obesity.[32] Obese children are also more likely to develop asthma.[33]

Obesity is the most significant risk factor for type 2 diabetes, a disease once called "adult onset diabetes" because it occurred almost exclusively in adults until childhood obesity started to rise substantially. The number of hospitalizations for type 2 diabetes among Americans in their 20s has gone up substantially, for example.[34] A 2001 study found that more than 75% of children ages 10 and over with type 2 diabetes were obese.[35] Type 2 diabetes occurs more frequently among some racial and ethnic minority groups, and rates among American Indians are particularly high.[36]

In addition to the physical health consequences, severely obese children report a lower health-related quality of life (a measure of their physical, emotional, educational, and social well-being) In fact, one study found that they have a similar quality of life as children diagnosed with cancer.[37] Childhood obesity is a highly stigmatized condition, often associated with low self-esteem, and obese children are more likely than non-obese children to feel sad, lonely, and nervous.[38] Obesity during childhood is also associated with some psychiatric disorders, including depression and binge-eating disorder, which may both contribute to and be adversely impacted by obesity.[39]

What Causes Obesity?

Early Life

A child's risk of becoming obese may even begin before birth Pregnant women who use tobacco, gain excessive weight, or have diabetes give birth to children who have an increased risk of being obese during their preschool years.[40] Furthermore, although the evidence is not conclusive,[41] rapid weight gain in early infancy has been shown to predict obesity later in life.[42] Racial and ethnic differences in obesity may also be partly explained by differences in risk factors during the prenatal period and early life.[43]

Studies show that early influences can affect obesity rates The increased occurrence of obesity among children of obese parents suggests a genetic component.[44] Multiple twin and adoption studies also indicate a strong genetic component to obesity.[45] However, genes associated with obesity were present in the population prior to the current epidemic; genes only account for susceptibility to obesity and generally contribute to obesity only when other influences are at work Genetic susceptibility to obesity is significantly shaped by the environment.[46] In addition to genetic factors, recent research has focused on other factors, such as maternal nutrition, environmental toxins, and the prenatal environment, which may shape later risk for childhood obesity.

Environmental Factors during Childhood

There have been major changes in Americans' lifestyles over the last 30 years, as childhood obesity rates have been rising. This includes what and where we eat Given the pace of modern life, Americans now consume more fast-food and sugar-sweetened beverages, eat outside the home more frequently,[47] and spend less time enjoying family meals In addition, prepared and processed food is easily accessible and inexpensive. These items are also heavily promoted, as evidenced in a Federal Trade Commission (FTC) report revealing that at least $1 6 billion is spent annually on food advertising directed to children and adolescents.[48] All this adds up to poor eating habits For example, 13% of the daily caloric intake for 12-19 year-olds now comes from sugar-sweetened beverages.[49]

At the same time, adults and children alike are getting less physical activity. Some schools have cut back on activities like physical education and recess, in part due to budget pressures at the state and local level. And children are increasingly driven to school by car or bus, rather than walking or biking. [50] In part, these shifts in transportation reflect changes in community design. Physical activity is higher in more "connected" communities that provide safe and reliable access to public transportation, as well as other forms of active transport like biking and walking. [51]

Meanwhile, "screen time" has increased, including television viewing, which is directly associated with childhood and adult obesity.[52] Among children, watching television or time spent on computers or gaming systems takes away from engaging in physical activity like organized sports or informal playing. It also has a more harmful effect on healthy eating habits; as children watch television, they are more likely to snack, including on the foods advertised.[53] In addition, screen time has been associated with children getting less and poorer quality sleep,[54] and insufficient sleep has been linked to a heightened risk of obesity.[55]

What Can We Do?

While additional studies to identify the precise causes of obesity will be useful, we do not need to wait to identify specific actions that we can take as a society to prevent obesity. There are many examples of effective therapies for diseases whose cause has not been fully identified. For example, remission rates of acute lymphocytic leukemia in children have been dramatically improved over the last 20 years, although the causes of the disease remain uncertain.

No single action alone will reverse the childhood obesity epidemic, although there is no question that improving eating habits and increasing physical activity are two critical strategies. As with tobacco prevention and control, comprehensive, multi-sectoral approaches are needed to address the many behavioral risk factors associated with obesity.[56] These risk factors fall into three general categories: (1) material incentives, such as the cost of food or the desire to avoid poor health; (2) social norms, such as the nutritional and physical activity habits of friends and family, which influence us greatly; and (3) the broader environment, such as whether grocery stores and playgrounds are nearby or far away Changes in each of these risk factors are possible. For example, with sound information, parents and caregivers will be able to seek out the most nutritious foods to improve their children's health; changes in social norms can be brought about through movements such as the successful seatbelt buckling campaigns of the late 20th century; and changes can be made in the broader environment by eliminating "food deserts" or "playground deserts. "

In many parts of the country, we already have a head start, and initiatives that are already underway will provide instructive lessons. Comprehensive, community-wide efforts to reduce obesity have recently been initiated by both the public and private sectors. The American Recovery and Reinvestment Act of 2009 included $1 billion in funding for prevention and wellness investments, more than half of which was directed to prevention strategies to reduce tobacco use and obesity rates. Specifically, $373 million supported direct community-based interventions and $120 million supported state-based efforts in all 50 states and 25 communities in urban, rural, and tribal areas. Funds to support comprehensive strategies were awarded to states in February and to communities in March. The recently-enacted Patient Protection and Affordable Care Act, as amended by the Health Care and Education Affordability Reconciliation Act (collectively referred to as the "Affordable Care Act") provides for additional investments in chronic disease and improving public health, which could include community-based prevention strategies In addition, the philanthropic sector has been leading the way with stepped-up, focused investments. For example, the Robert Wood Johnson Foundation has created a "Healthy Kids, Healthy Communities" initiative that is funding 50 communities to implement strategies to prevent childhood obesity,[57] and the California Endowment recently launched a large-scale "Building Healthy Communities" project in 14 communities that will include a focus on childhood obesity prevention. [58]

Reducing childhood obesity does not have to be a costly endeavor, however. And indeed, in many communities it simply cannot be Times are tough, and federal, state, local, and family budgets are all feeling squeezed. But a great deal can be accomplished without significant expenditures, and some steps may ultimately save money. [59] While many of the recommendations in this report will require additional public resources, creative strategies can also be used to redirect resources or make more effective use of existing investments.

In total, this report presents a series of 70 specific recommendations, many of which can be implemented right away Summarizing them broadly, they include:

- **Getting children a healthy start on life**, with good prenatal care for their parents; support for breastfeeding; adherence to limits on "screen time"; and quality child care settings with nutritious food and ample opportunity for young children to be physically active.
- **Empowering parents and caregivers** with simpler, more actionable messages about nutritional choices based on the latest *Dietary Guidelines for Americans*; improved labels on food and menus that provide clear information to help make healthy choices for children; reduced marketing of unhealthy products to children; and improved health care services, including BMI measurement for all children.
- **Providing healthy food in schools**, through improvements in federally-supported school lunches and breakfasts; upgrading the nutritional quality of other foods sold in schools; and improving nutrition education and the overall school environment.
- **Improving access to healthy, affordable food**, by eliminating "food deserts" in urban and rural America; lowering the relative prices of healthier foods; developing or reformulating food products to be healthier; and reducing the incidence of hunger, which has been linked to obesity.
- **Getting children more physically active**, through quality physical education, recess, and other opportunities in and after school; addressing aspects of the "built environment" that make it difficult for children to walk or bike safely in their

communities; and improving access to safe parks, playgrounds, and indoor and outdoor recreational facilities.

Many of these recommendations are for activities to be undertaken by federal agencies. All such activities are subject to budgetary constraints, including the weighing of priorities and available resources by the Administration in formulating its annual budget and by Congress in legislating appropriations.

How Will We Know We Have Succeeded?

Our goal is to solve the problem of childhood obesity in a generation Achieving that goal will mean returning to the expected levels in the population, before this epidemic began. That means ***returning to a childhood obesity rate of just 5% by 2030***. Achieving this goal will require "bending the curve" fairly quickly, so that by 2015, there will be a 2 5% reduction in each of the current rates of overweight and obese children, and by 2020, a 5% reduction. Our progress can be charted through the CDC's annual National Health and Nutrition Examination Survey (NHANES), which is aggregated every two years.

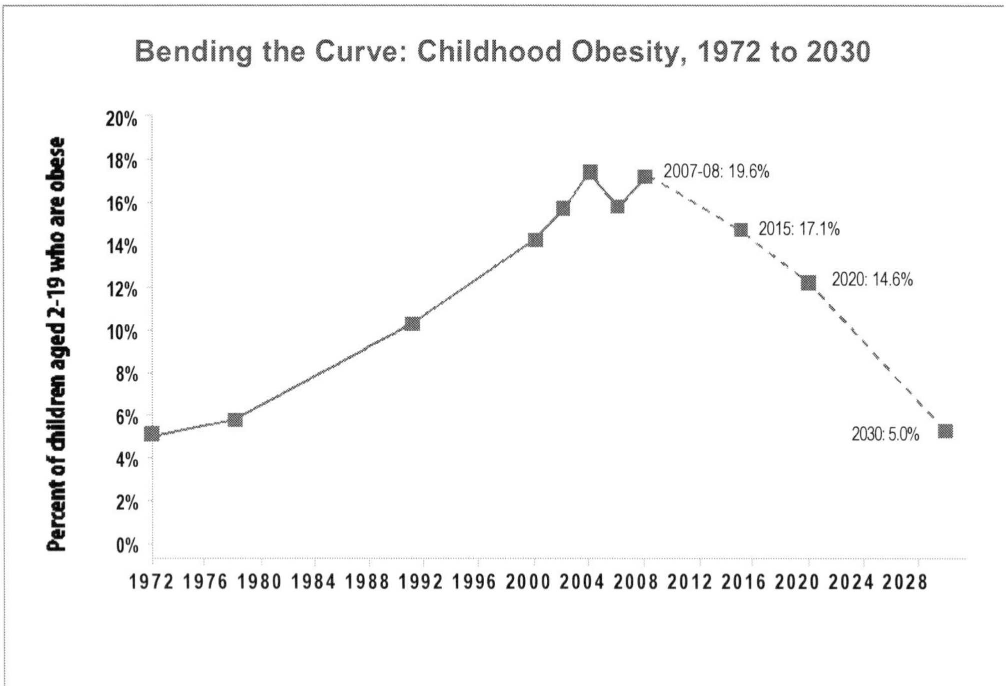

Source: CDC, National Center for Health Statistics, National Health and Nutrition Examination Surveys. Note: Obesity is defined as BMI ≥ gender- and weight-specific 95th percentile from the 2000 CDC Growth Charts.

In addition to monitoring the overall trends in childhood obesity, two key indicators will show the progress achieved:

1. **The number of children eating a healthy diet**, measured by those who follow the most recent, science-based *Dietary Guidelines for Americans (Dietary Guidelines).* We can monitor our progress through the U S Department of Agriculture's (USDA) Healthy Eating Index (HEI), which reflects the intake of 12 dietary components: total fruit (including juice); whole fruit (not juice); total vegetables; dark green and orange vegetables and legumes; total grains; whole grains; milk products; meat and beans; oils; saturated fat; sodium; and calories from solid fats and added sugars USDA generally regards a score of at least 80 out of 100 points as reflecting a healthy diet. Currently, the average child scores a 55 9 on the H EI. [60] To achieve a score of 80 for the average child by 2030, the average child should score 65 by 2015, and 70 by 2020 Two indicators should be monitored particularly closely:
   - **Less added sugar in children's diets.** Children today consume a substantial amount of added sugars through a whole range of products. Using existing data sources, CDC's National Center for Health Statistics can determine how much added sugar children are currently consuming. Targets for reducing added sugar will then need to be established that track the overall goal of driving obesity rates down to 5% by 2030.
   - **More fruits and vegetables.** Currently, children and adolescents consume far lower quantities of fruits and vegetables than recommended in the *Dietary Guidelines*. On average, children consumed only 64% of the recommended level of fruit and 46% of the recommended level of vegetables in 2003-04. Average fruit consumption should increase to 75% of the recommended level by 2015, 85% by 2020, and 100% by 2030; vegetable consumption should increase to 60% of recommended levels by 2015, 75% by 2020, and 100% by 2030.
2. **The number of children meeting current physical activity guidelines**. Right now, the only regular survey that shows whether children are meeting the Physical Activity Guidelines is limited to high school students, and regular data on younger children is not available. Resources will have to be redirected to develop a survey instrument that can provide a full picture of physical activity levels among children of all ages. Once baseline data is available, targets for improving the level of physical activity among children will need to be established that track the overall goal of driving obesity rates down to 5% by 2030.

Additional benchmarks of success, tied to specific recommendations in this report, are included throughout.The Healthy People goals set every decade by experts convened by the U.S. Department of Health and Human Services will provide additional, complementary opportunities to measure our progress in helping children achieve and maintain a healthy weight.

Monitoring our progress and the impact of our interventions, so that we know what is working and what strategies or tactics need to be adjusted, will be critically important. This is not an easy challenge, but it is one that we can solve as a society, and within a generation.

I. EARLY CHILDHOOD

Studies show that approximately one in five children are overweight or obese by the time they reach their 6th birthday,[61] and over half of obese children become overweight at or before age two. [62] Even babies are affected Between 1980 and 2001, the prevalence of overweight infants under six months almost doubled, from 3 4% to 5 9%. [63] More can and must be done to ensure our youngest children begin life on a healthy path.

This chapter provides recommendations for reducing the risk of obesity in the early years of a child's life by:

- strengthening prenatal care;
- promoting breastfeeding;
- evaluating the impact of chemical influences in the environment;
- reducing "screen time;" and
- improving the quality of our nation's child care settings so they can consistently support our children's healthy development.

A. Prenatal Care

Mothers' pre-conception weight and weight gain during pregnancy are two of the most important prenatal determinants of childhood obesity. Several factors may influence the association of maternal weight and weight gain during pregnancy with long-term child health outcomes. These factors include maternal and paternal BMI, maternal smoking during pregnancy, blood sugar levels during pregnancy, fetal growth, birth weight, and infant feeding practices.[64]

Higher maternal weight is a risk factor for gestational diabetes or related conditions during pregnancy. Children born to mothers who had diabetes during pregnancy are at higher risk of being overweight and having gestational and type 2 diabetes. In a study of low-income children, there was a association between maternal BMI in the first trimester and the probability of being overweight at 2, 3, and 4 years of age.

Recent findings suggest that very low birth weight and very high birth weight are both associated with childhood obesity. Although the link between very high birth weight and childhood obesity is studied more, the link between low birth weight and obesity may be the result of accelerated growth immediately after birth. Babies who were "deprived of nutrition" before birth may be primed for accelerated growth after birth when exposed to a rich nutrient environment (which often consists of infant formula).[65] This rapid growth in the first few months and even perhaps the first days of postnatal life, are associated with increased risk of children being overweight.[66]

Maternal smoking during early pregnancy is associated with a 500% greater risk of obesity at age 5, and a 260% greater risk at ages 9-10.[67] The duration of smoking while pregnant and number of cigarettes smoked per day are both associated with increases in rates of childhood obesity.[68] Maternal smoking is linked to low intrauterine growth, which can be associated with accelerated postnatal growth and childhood obesity. Notably, the recently-enacted Affordable Care Act requires coverage of counseling and pharmacotherapy for cessation of tobacco use for pregnant women in Medicaid, with no cost-sharing for these services, effective October 1.[69]

To improve children's health, the Surgeon General recommends promoting effective prenatal counseling about: maternal weight gain; breastfeeding; the relationship between obesity and diabetes; and avoiding alcohol, tobacco, and drug use during pregnancy.[70] Recent clinical trials indicate that weight gain can be modified by prenatal counseling.[71] Currently, however, only about 30% of pregnant women receive appropriate counseling and guidance from a medical professional on how to achieve recommended weight goals during pregnancy.[72]

Higher maternal weight gain during pregnancy is also associated with excess maternal weight retained afte childbirth.[73] A higher BMI after childbirth can be a health risk for the mother but also sets the stage for a higher pre-pregnancy weight in future pregnancies.

A more complete picture of maternal and child weight is needed to monitor these trends and better inform policymakers and health professionals.

Recommendations

Recommendation 1.1: Pregnant women and women planning a pregnancy should be informed of the importance of conceiving at a healthy weight and having a healthy weight gain during pregnancy, based on the relevant recommendations of the Institute of Medicine. Specifically, health care providers, as well as Federal, state, and local agencies, medical societies, and organizations that serve pregnant women or those planning pregnancies should provide information concerning the importance of conceiving at a normal BMI and having a healthy weight gain during pregnancy. Those who provide primary and prenatal care to women should offer them counseling on dietary intake and physical activity that is tailored to their life circumstances. In many cases, conceiving at a normal BMI will require some weight loss.

TEXT4BABY: PROVIDING HEALTH TIPS TO PREGNANT WOMEN AND NEW PARENTS

Text4baby, an educational program of the U.S. Department of Health and Human Services and the National Healthy Mothers, Healthy Babies Coalition, is a free mobile information service that provides pregnant women and new parents with health tips to help them give their babies the best possible start in life.

Recommendation 1.2: Education and outreach efforts about prenatal care should be enhanced through creative approaches that take into account the latest in technology and communications. Partners in this effort could include companies that develop technology-based communications tools, as well as companies that market products and services to pregnant women or prospective parents.

Benchmarks of Success

A higher percentage of women conceiving at a normal BMI, and at an appropriate gestational weight gain during pregnancy, based on the Institute of Medicine's gestational weight guidelines.[74] To measure this, HHS should redirect existing resources to prioritize routine surveillance of weight gain during pregnancy and postpartum weight retention on a nationally representative sample of women and to report the results by pre-pregnancy BMI (including all classes of obesity), age, racial/ethnic group, and socioeconomic status.

Some states also collect maternal and child weight information on birth certificates, and states should be encouraged to work with HHS to ensure that a complete set of data is collected. The 2003 version of the U.S. Standard Certificate of Live Birth includes fields for maternal pre-pregnancy weight, height, weight at delivery, and age at the last measured weight, facilitating improved public health surveillance.[75] By 2007, 24 states adopted this form, representing an estimated 60% of all births.[76] States should strive for 100% completion of fields related to maternal weight and height, as well as share data to provide a full national picture and regional snapshots. HHS should work with the remaining states to encourage adoption of the updated birth certificate form. The President's FY2011 Budget includes increased resources for all States to have an electronic birth record in 2011.

As an interim step, prenatal counseling rates can be measured as a proxy. The Pregnancy Risk Assessment Monitoring System (PRAMS) is a surveillance project of the CDC and state health departments. PRAMS collects state-specific, population-based data on maternal attitudes and experiences before, during, and shortly after pregnancy, including information on prenatal counseling, cigarette use, alcohol use, breastfeeding, and pre-conception health (including height and weight). PRAMS will be revised to capture prenatal counseling on appropriate weight gain.

B. Breastfeeding

Children who are breastfed are at reduced risk of obesity.77 Studies have found that the likelihood of obesity is 22% lower among children who were breastfed.[78] The strongest effects were observed among adolescents, meaning that the obesity-reducing benefits of breastfeeding extend many years into a child's life. Another study determined that the risk of becoming overweight was reduced by 4% for each month of breastfeeding.[79] This effect plateaued after nine months of breastfeeding.

Despite these health benefits, although most (74%) babies start out breastfeeding, within three months, two-thirds (67%) have already received formula or other supplements. By six months of age, only 43% are still breastfeeding at all, and less than one quarter (23%) are breastfed at least 12 months.[80] In addition, there is a disparity between the prevalence of breastfeeding among non-Hispanic black infants and those in other racial or ethnic groups. For instance, a recent CDC study showed a difference of greater than 20 percentage points in 13 states.[81]

The protective effect of breastfeeding likely results from a combination of factors. First, infant formula contains nearly twice as much protein per serving as breast milk. This excess protein may stimulate insulin secretion in an unhealthy way.[82] Second, the biological response to breast milk differs from that of formula. When feeding a baby, the mother's milk prompts the baby's liver to release a protein that helps regulate metabolism.[83] Feeding formula instead of breast milk increases the baby's concentrations of insulin in his or her blood, prolongs insulin response,[84] and, even into childhood, is associated with unfavorable concentrations of leptin, a hormone that inhibits appetite and controls body fatness.[85] Despite the well-known health benefits of breastfeeding and the preference of most pregnant women to breastfeed,[86] numerous barriers make breastfeeding difficult. For first-time mothers, breastfeeding can be challenging, even for those who intend to breastfeed. For those who have less clear intent to breastfeed, cultural, social, or structural challenges can prevent breastfeeding initiation or continuation. For example, immediately after birth, many babies are unnecessarily given formula and separated from their mothers, making it harder to start and practice breastfeeding. Also, hospital staff are often insufficiently trained in breastfeeding support.

The Joint Commission on the Accreditation of Hospitals, the body that accredits hospitals and health care organizations for most State Medicaid and Medicare reimbursement, now expects hospitals to track and improve their rates of exclusive breastfeeding. Hospitals that meet specific criteria for optimal breastfeeding-related maternity care are designated as "Baby Friendly" by Baby-Friendly U.S.A. This non-governmental organization has been named by the U.S. Committee for UNICEF as the designating authority for UNICEF/WHO standards in the United States. Currently only 3% of births in America occur in Baby-Friendly facilities.[87]

While breastfeeding could be far more widespread than it is today, it is not a viable alternative for all mothers and babies. Specific guidance and support options should also be made available for those who cannot breastfeed. Parents and caregivers of babies also may benefit from guidance about when to start feeding them solid foods, since early introduction of solids (prior to six months) increases the risk for childhood obesity.[88]

Workplace and Child Care Accommodations

Research has demonstrated that support is essential for helping mothers establish and continue breastfeeding as they return to work or school and make use of child care services.89 Many women return to work soon after their baby's birth, yet 75% of employers do not offer accommodations for them to breastfeed or express milk at work.[90]

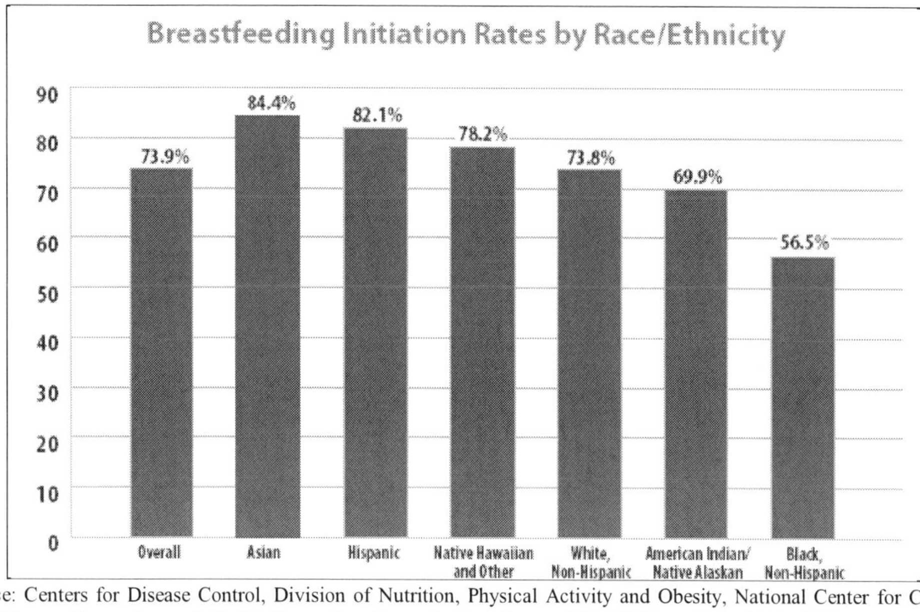

Source: Centers for Disease Control, Division of Nutrition, Physical Activity and Obesity, National Center for Chronic Disease Prevention and Health Promotion. Breastfeeding Among U.S. Children Born 1999–2006, CDC National Immunization Survey.

Changes are underway, however. Following the lead of states whose laws requiring employers to make accommodations, the recently-enacted Affordable Care Act requires employers to provide a reasonable break time and a place for breastfeeding mothers to express milk for one year after their child's birth.[91] Employers with fewer than 50 employees are not subject to these requirements if compliance would impose an undue hardship. The location cannot be a bathroom, and must be shielded from view and free from intrusion from co-workers and the public. The return on investment of companies that assist breastfeeding employees through appropriate support and accommodations is well-documented. Companies benefit through better employee retention, lower health care costs, and better work attendance.[92]

Support for breastfeeding in child care settings is important as well. Among women whose infants are cared for outside the home, irrespective of their intent to breastfeed, those who report better support for breastfeeding from early learning settings (such as refrigerated storage for breast milk, a commitment to feed it to the child, or privacy space for on-site breastfeeding) are more likely to breastfeed longer.[93]

Support Programs

In many communities, role models for breastfeeding are rare, and new mothers do not know where to turn for breastfeeding assistance. Volunteer networks of experienced breastfeeding mothers such as the La Leche League provide help for some mothers, but networks like this are not available in many communities. According to the CDC's annual State Breastfeeding Report Card, there were 34 breastfeeding

support groups per 100,000 live births in 2009, which means about one support group for every 3000 new babies. Peer support programs, such as the Peer Counselor program delivered as part of the Special Supplemental Nutrition Program for Women, Infants and Children (WIC), provide counseling skills, training, and support to experienced breastfeeding mothers so they can effectively support new mothers. Recently, federal funds were provided to further expand the availability of peer counseling in local WIC clinics. Prenatal counseling on breastfeeding can also have positive impacts on breastfeeding rates,[94] and pre- and postnatal intervention together with peer counseling is most effective.[95]

Recommendations

Recommendation 1.3: Hospitals and health care providers should use maternity care practices that empower new mothers to breastfeed, such as the Baby-Friendly hospital standards. Hospitals and health care providers should routinely provide evidence-based maternity care that empowers parents to make informed infant feeding decisions as active participants in their care, and improves new mothers' ability to breastfeed successfully. Examples of specific practices and policies include: skin-to-skin contact between the mother and her baby; teaching mothers how to breastfeed; and early and frequent breastfeeding opportunities.

Hospitals, health care providers, and health insurers should also help ensure that new mothers receive proper information and support on breastfeeding when they are released from the hospital.

Recommendation 1.4: Health care providers and insurance companies should provide information to pregnant women and new mothers on breastfeeding, including the availability of educational classes, and connect pregnant women and new mothers to breastfeeding support programs to help them make an informed infant feeding decision.

Recommendation 1.5: Local health departments and community-based organizations, working with health care providers, insurance companies, and others should develop peer support programs that empower pregnant women and mothers to get the help and support they need from other mothers who have breastfed. Peer support networks should exist in all communities across the country, allowing all new mothers to easily identify and obtain help from trained breastfeeding peer counselors. Community organizations can foster the creation of peer support networks through expansion of programs like the WIC Breastfeeding Peer Counseling program. They can work with local breastfeeding coalitions to ensure existence of other peer support networks, such as La Leche League groups or Nursing Mothers Councils. They can also foster the creation of mother-to-mother support groups in community health centers and advertise these groups, particularly as part of the hospital discharge process.

Early Head Start (EHS) programs that enroll pregnant women, including pregnant teenagers, can also support community breastfeeding networks. EHS can provide home visits and reach out to pregnant and breastfeeding mothers to encourage and support breastfeeding, including by providing professional and peer opportunities to disseminate information and provide on-going support. Funding for evidence-based home visitation programs in the recently-enacted Affordable Care Act[96] will complement this program.

Private companies, including those that market baby products, can also help support and promote these types of community supports for mothers.

Recommendation 1.6: Early childhood settings should support breastfeeding. Child care centers and providers, health care providers, and government agencies should provide accurate information about the storage and handling of breast milk. They should also make sure child care employees and providers know how to store, handle, and feed breast milk, and understand the importance of breastfeeding.

Benchmarks of Success

An increase in breastfeeding rates. Several government sources provide statistics on breastfeeding rates. The most comprehensive source of information is the National Immunization Survey, which provides annual national, state, and selected urban-area estimates of breastfeeding initiation, duration, and exclusivity. In addition to questions on breastfeeding, the survey asks about the introduction of infant formula and other supplementary foods. As noted above, according to the survey, currently 30% of babies age nine months or younger are breastfed. This should increase by 5% every two years, so that by 2015, half of babies are breastfed for at least nine months.

C. Chemical Exposures

In addition to fetal "over-nutrition" or "under-nutrition," it is possible that developmental exposure to endocrine disrupting chemicals (EDCs) or other chemicals plays a role in the development of diabetes and childhood obesity. Some scientists have coined the term "obesogens" for chemicals that they believe may promote weight gain and obesity. Such chemicals may promote obesity by increasing the number of fat cells, changing the amount of calories burned at rest, altering energy balance, and altering the body's mechanisms for appetite and satiety. Fetal and infant exposure to such chemicals may result in more weight gain per food consumed and also possibly less weight loss per amount of energy expended. The health effects of these chemicals during fetal and infant development may persist throughout life, long after the exposures occur.[97]

Research on such chemicals suggests that the origins of obesity may lie not only in well-established risk factors such as diet and exercise, but also in the interplay between genes and the fetal and early postnatal environment. The National Institute of Environmental Health Sciences, the Environmental Protection Agency (EPA), and other research organizations have been working to understand the developmental origins of obesity and other diseases. Their activities have helped reveal the links between environmental chemicals and obesity and diabetes, providing a sufficient base of evidence to warrant future research efforts in this area.

This issue could also be investigated further by the President's Task Force on Environmental Health Risks and Safety Risks to Children, led by HHS and EPA. An increased understanding of chemical toxicity also adds strength to the existing recommendations for parents to avoid microwaving baby bottles or plastic containers that are not explicitly stated by the manufacturer as safe for use in microwaving.[98] Government should work closely with industries to translate this emerging science into programs that supports product reformulation (for example, of plastic containers) as appropriate.

Recommendations

Recommendation 1.7: Federal and State agencies conducting health research should prioritize research into the effects of possibly obesogenic chemicals. As the research becomes clearer, reducing harmful exposures may require outreach to communities and medical providers, and could also entail regulatory action.

Benchmarks of Success

A stronger knowledge of chemical exposures that may be related to obesity. Emerging research will guide the direction of future intervention strategies for which progress metrics can then be developed. The necessary research will control the timeline for at least the first 4-5 years. After that time, while research efforts will continue, there may be sufficient information to develop strategies to eliminate exposures identified as obesogenic.

D. Screen Time

The American Academy of Pediatrics (AAP) recommends that children two years old and under should not be exposed to television, and children over age two should limit daily media exposure to only 1-2 hours of quality programming.[99] In contrast to these recommendations, one study found that 43% of children under age two watch television daily, and 26% have a television in their room.[100]

Preschool aged children are also watching more television than recommended by the AAP. Ninety percent of children ages 4-6 use screen media for an average of two hours per day. Over 40% of children in this age group have a television in their bedroom, a third have a portable DVD player, and a third have a portable handheld video game player. Children from lower income families and children of color spend more time watching television and are more likely to live in a home where it is left on most of the time.[101]

Studies show an association between television viewing and risk of being overweight in preschool children, independent of socio-demographic factors. Specifically, for each additional hour of television viewing, the odds ratio of children having a BMI greater than the 85th percentile was 1.06.[102] Having a television in the bedroom had a stronger association, with an odds ratio of 1.31. One study noted that preschool children who watched television for more than two hours a day were more likely to be overweight than children who watched television two hours or less daily.[103]

Television viewing is also linked to dietary intake. Another study found that television exposure was correlated with fast-food consumption in preschool children, even after adjusting for a variety of socio-demographic and socio-environmental factors.[104]

Recommendations

***Recommendation 1.8: The AAP guidelines on screen time should be made more available to parents, and young children should be encouraged to spend less time using digital media and more time being physically active*.** Health care provider visits and meetings with teachers and early learning providers are an opportunity to give guidance and information to parents and their children.

Recommendation 1.9: The AAP guidelines on screen time should be made more available in early childhood settings. Early childhood settings should be encouraged to adopt standards consistent with AAP recommendations not to expose children two years of age and under to television, as well as to limit media exposure for older children by treating it as a special occasion activity rather than a daily event.

E. Early Care and Education

More than 3.5 million children under age five are cared for in child care centers, and many more are cared for through less formal arrangements while a parent works.[105] Children in child care centers spent an average of 33 hours a week in those settings.[106] Parents and child care providers are sharing the responsibility for a large and growing number of children during important developmental years. Early childhood settings, including both child care centers and informal care, present a tremendous opportunity to prevent obesity by making an impact at a pivotal phase in children's lives.

Physical Activity

Young children need opportunities to be physically active through play and other activities. Physical activity assists children in obtaining and improving fine and gross motor skill development, coordination, balance and control, hand-eye coordination, strength, dexterity, and flexibility—all of which are necessary for children to reach developmental milestones.

Preschool years, in particular, are crucial for obesity prevention due to the timing of the development of fat tissue, which typically occurs from ages 3-7. During these preschool years, children's BMI typically reaches its lowest point and then increases gradually through adolescence and most of adulthood. However, if this BMI increase begins before ages 4 to 6, research has suggested that children face a greater risk of obesity in adulthood.[107]

Features of the child care center environment, including policies regarding activity and provider training, as well as the presence of portable and fixed play equipment, influence the amount of physical activity children engage in while at child care.[108]

Healthy Eating

Eating well is equally important for the healthy development of young children, and research has shown that public programs can improve the nutritional quality of the food consumed in child care settings. Children in early childhood settings who are served by USDA's Child and Adult Care Food Program (CACFP) eat healthier food than children who bring meals and snacks from home.109 A comparison of meal quality among licensed early learning sites in California found that children eating meals provided in Head Start had the highest meal quality scores, followed by those eating in non-Head Start under CACFP. Meal quality scores were higher among center-based versus home-based facilities.[110]

Many programs have already seized the opportunity to provide healthier foods and have implemented evidence-informed initiatives that encourage healthy eating and fun, developmentally-appropriate physical activity. Still, there is room for improvement.[111] Empirically-based and practice-tested strategies for improving these settings have been identified and provide a basis for the recommendations outlined in this chapter. Through concerted and coordinated effort at the Federal, state, and local levels, today's early learning settings can support healthy weight through the development of good habits for nutrition, physical activity, and screen time.

Each state creates and enforces its own child care licensing standards, as well as other program standards for center-based and family child care homes. Not all child care facilities are required to be licensed in order to legally operate within a state, but they must meet some basic requirements. A recent review of state child care regulations by researchers at the Duke University School of Medicine, based on ten expert-derived healthy eating model regulations, found that states had an average of 3.7 healthy eating regulations for child care centers and 2 9 for family child care homes. No state had all ten model regulations States had particularly few regulations relating to physical activity and screen time. [112]

Workforce qualifications and training requirements for child care providers also vary widely from state to state. Many states are now implementing Professional Development Registries and other methods to better track and document the providers' training sessions. They are also implementing observation and feedback opportunities to understand if training is being applied in the classroom. To incorporate recommended nutrition, physical activity, and screen standards into their curricula, Federal agencies and states can partner with national organizations such as the National Association of Child Care Resource and Referral Agencies (NACCRRA), the National Association for the Education of Young Children (NAEYC), and the National Head Start Association (NHSA), as well as community colleges and other training providers.

Parents are often unaware of quality elements when choosing child care and early education settings, including the importance of nutrition, physical activity, and screen time limits provided in these settings, and they can find it difficult to get this information. Quality Rating and Improvement Systems (QRISs) are State systems that rate the quality of early child care settings (which can include Pre-K, Head Start, child care, and others) based on a clear, common set of criteria. These rating systems can provide parents with reliable, consistent information that can help them make informed decisions.

INNOVATIVE EARLY CHILDHOOD PROGRAMS

There are several evidence-informed initiatives and interventions for early childhood settings to combat childhood obesity, including:

- *I am Moving, I am Learning,* a proactive approach to childhood obesity in preschool classrooms that seeks to increase moderate to vigorous physical activity every day, improve the quality of movement activities intentionally planned and facilitated by adults, and promote healthy food choices. This approach is implemented by Head Start and has been adopted by some other child care programs as well.
- *Nutrition and Physical Activity Self-Assessment for Child Care (NAP SACC),* an assessment tool for child care settings, which uses an organizational assessment of 14 areas of nutrition and physical activity policy, practices and environments to identify the strengths and limitations of the child care facility. NAP SACC also includes goal setting and action planning, continuing education and skill building for providers.
- *Nemours Program:* Delaware, under the leadership of Nemours, an integrated child health system, launched a statewide, multi-sector program to combat childhood obesity that includes changes in child care licensing to set healthy eating and physical activity standards, along with technical assistance, training and practical toolkits to help providers implement the standards. The new standards apply to all licensed center and family day care providers, impacting 54,000 children.

Recommendations

Recommendation 1.10: The Federal government, incorporating input from health care providers and other stakeholders, should provide clear, actionable guidance to states, providers, and families on how to increase physical activity, improve nutrition, and reduce screen time in early child care settings.

Recommendation 1.11: States should be encouraged to strengthen licensing standards and Quality Rating and Improvement Systems to support good program practices regarding nutrition, physical activity, and screen time in early education and child care settings.

Both federal guidance and state policies and practices may be drawn from:

- The guidelines for Out-of-Home Child Care Programs that will be outlined in the soon-tobe released third edition of *Caring for our Children: National Health and Safety Performance Standards.*[113] These nationally recognized standards include health and safety practices such as physical activity, nutrition, and limited screen time for children from birth to age 12 in all types of early childhood settings.
- The National Association for Sport and Physical Education (NASPE) recommendation that all children in full-day child care are provided at least 60 minutes of structured and unstructured physical activity per day. Others have recommended that infants be provided opportunities for gross motor activity, and should not be unnecessarily confined.
- The revised Head Start Program Performance Standards, which include recommendations for health, nutrition, and physical environments.

Recommendation 1.12: The Federal government should look for opportunities in all early childhood programs it funds (such as the Child and Adult Care Food Program at USDA, the Child Care and Development Block Grant, Head Start, military child care, and Federal employee child care) to base policies and practices on current scientific evidence related to child nutrition and physical activity, and seek to improve access to these programs.

Benchmarks of Success

An increased number of states will adopt more stringent licensing standards that include nutrition, physical activity, and screen time that align with *Caring for our Children: National Health and Safety Performance Standards, 3rd edition* and coordinate across systems with Pre-K, Head Start, and child care. New or enhanced data sources may be needed to monitor progress in this area.

II. Empowering Parents and Caregivers

Fundamentally, parents and caregivers are responsible for their children's health and development. They instill and promote certain values, reward or reinforce specific behaviors, and shape choices that form life-long healthy habits. Each day, parents and caregivers make decisions on food selection, eating patterns, physical activity, and sedentary habits like television viewing. Children learn from the choices adults make. Often it is an entire family that experiences being overweight or obese.

Changes in the food and social environment over the past 20 years have made parents' and caregivers' roles in promoting health more challenging. Parents and caregivers want to provide good nutrition and regular physical activity, but often lack information that is clearly understandable and actionable. Communities, businesses, health care providers, and governments can play a supportive role in providing helpful information and fostering environments that support parents' and caregivers' healthy choices. For information to be useful to busy and overworked parents and caregivers, both the "what" and the "how" to deliver information must be considered. With a myriad of messages about what to eat and how to be active, the consistent delivery of specific, unambiguous, and actionable messages is critically important. In addition, the broader environment—including confusing claims or labels on food packages and marketing campaigns—can become a serious obstacle, by making unhealthy choices easy and healthy choices hard.

This chapter describes current and proposed initiatives to empower parents and caregivers by:

- making nutrition information useful,
- improving food marketing and labeling practices, and
- strengthening health care providers' role

A. Making Nutrition Information Useful

Good nutrition plays an essential role in overall health Healthy eating habits in childhood and adolescence are important for positive growth and development and can help children achieve and maintain a healthy weight. Today, the eating habits of many young people are inconsistent with the recommendations in the Federal *Dietary Guidelines for Americans (Dietary Guidelines*),[114] thus increasing the risk of obesity.

To assist parents and caregivers in establishing healthy eating habits for children, they should have greater access to the right tools and resources that increase nutritional knowledge and help them make healthier choices.

Dietary Guidelines for Americans and the Food Pyramid

The *Dietary Guidelines for Americans* provide science-based advice for individuals over age two to promote health and reduce the risk of major chronic diseases through diet and physical activity. HHS and USDA work in partnership to review and update these guidelines every five years, based on an analysis of scientific evidence. The current Dietary Guidelines, issued in 2005, encourage most. Americans to eat fewer calories, be more physically active, and make wiser food choices The 2010 Dietary Guidelines are under development, and will be released later this year.

> The **Dietary Guidelines** provide science-based advice about good dietary habits that can promote health and reduce the risk of major chronic disease.

The *Dietary Guidelines* are intended to be the primary source of dietary health information for policymakers, nutrition educators, and health providers, helping to inform nutrition research pri- orities, influence industry product development, and support education initiatives. They affect the decisions both private and public institutions make, and ultimately, they are meant to inform consumers, including parents and caregivers, about how to make healthy choices.

The *Dietary Guidelines* also form the basis of Federal nutrition policy. For example, they must be applied in menu planning in the National School Lunch Program (NSLP), in education materials used by the Supplemental Nutrition Assistance Program (SNAP, formerly called food stamps), and in the development of information on the Nutrition Facts panel that appears on food packages.

The Food Pyramid is an educational system developed by USDA to translate the *Dietary Guidelines* into food-based recommendations and applications for the public. The broader MyPyramid Food Guidance System provides educational resources, messages and personalized tips about nutrition and physical activity, and extensive online interactive healthy eating tools.

MyPyramid gov has reached millions of consumers, health professionals, and educators since it was launched in 2005, and is consistently one of the top five most popular federal web sites Despite its popularity and prominence, the Food Pyramid has been subject to significant criticism for failing to communicate effective, actionable messages to consumers, which many observers have suggested are critical in changing behavior. [115] The MyPyramid system is currently being studied for improvements.

In addition, the recently-enacted Affordable Care Act requires HHS, in consultation with private-sector experts, to maintain a website that provides science-based information to health care providers and consumers on guidelines for areas such as nutrition, regular exercise, and obesity reduction. The legislation also requires HHS to create a web-based prevention plan tool to help families make informed health decisions. [116] Parents and caregivers can also currently find information about nutrition and healthy eating at www.FruitsandVeggiesMatter gov and through the We Can childhood obesity prevention program developed by the National Institutes of Health (wecan nhlbi.nih.gov). Given the broad array of federal tools to help consumers make healthy choices, it is critical that these tools be developed and maintained in a manner that is coordinated and sending consistent messages.

Food Package Labeling

Parents and children need accurate, clear, and consistent information on food packages in order to choose healthier foods. At present, the main source of consistent information is the detailed Nutrition Facts panel on food packages, designed by the Food and Drug Administration (FDA) pursuant to the Nutrition Labeling and Education Act of 1990. USDA regulates the labeling of meat and poultry products, and currently requires the Nutrition Facts to be displayed on processed products USDA is in the process of requiring that the Nutrition Facts panel be displayed on other meat and poultry products, including ground beef and cuts of meat, as well. [117] According to recent FDA surveys, consumers are increasingly seeking nutrition information about the food they purchase.

The percent of the U.S. population that reports "often" reading a food label the first time they buy a product increased from 44% in 2002 to 54% in 2008. Of those that read food labels when purchasing a product for the first time in 2008, the food label was most often used to:

- See how high or low a food is in things like calories, salt, vitamins or fat (two-thirds of consumers).
- Get a general idea of the nutritional content of the food (over one-half of consumers).

Use of the Nutrition Facts nearly doubled in only four years, from 32% in 2004 to 52% in 2008. [118]

Nutritional or health claims on the front of food packages have also increased, but these claims are sometimes seen as misleading. An FDA survey found that only about half or less of Americans trust the claims on the front of food packages. [119] FDA has the authority to review scientific evidence for nutrient content and health claims on food packages before they are used, and is increasingly taking action to help prevent the spread of misinformation. FDA has taken action recently to address some of the inappropriate use of claims in food labeling.[120]

Despite its value and importance, the Nutrition Facts panel has been criticized as unduly detailed and complex. To make it easier for consumers to get information at a quick glance, FDA is currently investigating options for a standard, front-of package label. FDA is also working to update the Nutrition Facts panel based on new scientific information and consumer research.

"Spot the Block" Campaign

HHS has launched a program called "Spot the Block" to encourage children and caregivers to read the Nutrition Facts panel. They have recently launched an education campaign based on "Spot the Block" that targets African- American and Hispanic communities. HHS tested the "Spot the Block" program with the Cartoon Network and the research findings showed the program is effective in getting children to respond to the messages. Specifically, there were significant increases in:

- children who think the Nutrition Fact panel is important to them (+21%);
- the likelihood children would tell their friends to check the Nutrition Facts panel (+48%); and
- the perceived importance of knowing the serving sizes of the food they eat (+71%).

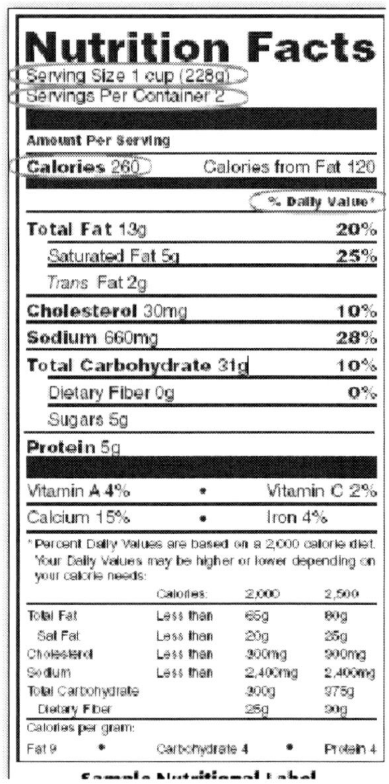

Serving sizes also play an important role. In 2005, FDA began the process of reviewing data to update the reference amounts used to determine serving sizes on food packages. A specific concern was the presentation of serving size information on packages that may contain multiple servings but could reasonably be consumed at one time. For example, a 20 ounce bottle of soda is currently labeled as having multiple servings, but is often consumed all at once. FDA is currently analyzing comments and food intake survey data to determine steps to take and how changes in serving size will impact updates to the Nutrition Facts panel.

Menu Labeling

The recently-enacted Affordable Care Act requires display of calorie counts by chain restaurants with 20 or more locations and vending machine operators with 20 or more machines.[121] Chain restaurants must also make available for customers, upon request, more detailed nutritional information such as sodium and sugars, and the menu or menu board must also include a clear statement indicating the availability of this information. Chain restaurants must display this information on menus, menu boards, self-service lines, and in drive-through lanes. Vending machines must provide a clear and noticeable statement disclosing the calorie counts near each item or the selection button. Restaurants, retail food establishments, and vending machine owners who are not subject to these requirements can voluntarily register with HHS to be subject to these requirements. New York City implemented a similar law prior to enactment of the Affordable Care Act, and early research indicates it may have favorably affected eating habits, although firm conclusions cannot yet be drawn.[122]

A recent study showed that both information and convenience can have a beneficial effect on how customers choose their meals. The study indicates that when presented with calorie information (how many calories are contained in each menu item) and a calorie recommendation (how many calories men and women of varying activity levels should consume), people on average order meals with significantly fewer calories. Indeed, the effect of providing this information reduced meals by almost 100 calories.[123] The study also showed that making healthier meal choices more convenient has a significant impact on consumption decisions. For example, if healthier options are featured on a menu page and other options require a more active choice, it is likely that fast-food customers will order lower calorie meals. This finding is consistent with other studies showing that changes in how and where food is located can help promote healthy choices, suggesting the effectiveness of possible changes like moving vending machines farther from school cafeterias or moving fruit next to cash registers.[124]

Research has also shown that plate size in restaurants or at home can make a significant difference in how much food is consumed,[125] and that portion sizes have grown substantially over time.[126] Eating dinner as a family is also associated with healthier eating.[127]

Recommendations

Recommendation 2.1: The Federal government, working with local communities, should dissemi-nate information about the 2010 Dietary Guidelines for Americans through simple, easily action-able messages for consumers and a next generation Food Pyramid. As HHS and USDA launch the updated Dietary Guidelines in late 2010, they should include simple advice and messages for consumers. Incorporating information about knowing daily caloric needs will be useful as menu labeling is implemented For example, these messages could include:

- Drink water instead of soda or juice with added sugar;
- Avoid foods that consist mainly of added sugars or fats;
- Eat more fruits, vegetables, whole grains, and lean proteins;
- Choose low-fat or fat-free dairy products (such as 1% or skim milk); and
- When possible, eat dinner together as a family.

Other important messages to share with parents include:

- The recommended amount of daily physical activity (one hour a day for children, as recommended by the companion *Physical Activity Guidelines for Americans);*
- The recommended amount of screen time; and
- The recommended amount of sleep (more than 10 5 hours a night for preschool-aged children and 12 hours for infants).[128]

Any specific messages should be coordinated with the scientific recommendations of the Dietary Guidelines Advisory Committee. They should also be coupled with practical tips for parents on how to make these changes in their children's lives. The tips should recognize the juggling act and time pressures that many parents and caregivers are facing. Suggestions for how to deliver these messages should also be sensitive to the risk of eating disorders among young people.

USDA and HHS should also research and disseminate information about the most effective ways to promote the Dietary Guidelines among children to impact their eating habits. This includes modernizing the "SNAP Ed" program, a nutrition education program for participants in SNAP (formerly known as food stamps), in a way that provides influential information to parents and caregivers. A recent study recommended that SNAP Ed be improved in a number of ways.[129]

Recommendation 2.2: The FDA and USDA's Food Safety and Inspection Service should collaborate with the food and beverage industry to develop and implement a standard system of nutrition labeling for the front of packages. The labeling system should be based on scientific research that assesses the formats people will notice, understand, and use to make healthy choices To complement this effort, FDA should address portion size and continue its work to prevent misleading claims on food packages.

Recommendation 2.3: Restaurants and vending machine operators subject to the new requirement in the Affordable Care Act should be encouraged to begin displaying calorie counts as soon as possible.

Recommendation 2.4: Restaurants should consider their portion sizes, improve children's menus, and make healthy options the default choice whenever possible. The improvements are particularly important since one-third of meals are consumed in restaurants,[130] including many meals eaten by children at fast-food establishments.

Benchmarks of Success

An increase in the number of parents who are better able to notice, understand, and use food labels. FDA collects data on use of nutrition labels by adult consumers in households with children through the Health and Diet Survey and will be looking for a steady increase in the percentage using the labels.

In addition, as noted earlier in this report, it will be critically important to monitor the overall health of children's diets and make steady progress toward improvements such as reducing added sugars and increasing fruit and vegetable consumption.

B. Food Marketing

Food marketing to children and adolescents is a big business. The Federal Trade Commission (FTC) estimates that, in 2006, food, beverage, and quick-serve restaurant companies spent more than $1.6 billion to promote their products to young people.[131] Children and adolescents are an important demographic for marketers for several reasons: (1) they are customers themselves; (2) they influence purchases made by parents and caregivers; and (3) they are the future adult market.[132] For many years, public health experts and others have argued that the marketing of energy-dense, low-nutrient food products to children and adolescents is one of many factors contributing to the obesity epidemic. While a causal link between marketing and increasing childhood obesity rates has yet to be firmly established,[133] research indicates that advertising can have a strong influence on children. Young children in particular have difficulty distinguishing between television programming content and advertising, or comprehending the purpose of advertising.[134] Older children, and even adults, are influenced by advertising too.

The marketing of food products can also be a powerful tool to drive the purchase of healthy products and to communicate important information about healthy eating choices. For example, one study found that children ages 3-5 preferred the taste of the same foods if they thought they were from McDonald's, rather than another source.[135] Key actors—from food and beverage companies, to restaurants, food retailers, trade associations, the media, government and others—all have an important role to play in creating a food marketing environment that supports, rather than undermines, the efforts of parents and other caregivers to encourage healthy eating among children and prevent obesity.

Current Climate, Recent Initiatives, and Industry Self-Regulation

Television advertising is the dominant form of marketing to both children and adolescents, comprising almost half of total youth-directed marketing expenditures according to the FTC.[136] However, food and beverage companies utilize a full range of other marketing techniques including print, internet advertising (such as advergames), product packaging, in-school marketing, cross-promotions, prizes and contests, and the use of popular licensed characters that appeal to children and adolescents.[137] Notably, many advertising campaigns are fully integrated, using common themes across multiple promotional platforms.[138]

The use of licensed characters to market foods to children is particularly effective and pervasive. Research conducted by the Sesame Street Workshop in 2005 found a strong influence of popular licensed characters on preschoolers' food preferences.[139] When preschoolers were asked if they would rather eat broccoli or a Hershey's chocolate bar, 78% of the children chose the chocolate bar and only 22% chose broccoli. When an Elmo sticker was placed on the broccoli, however, 50% of the children chose broccoli. Not surprisingly, food marketers' use of licensed characters in cross promotions targeting children has increased in recent years.[140] At the same time, the nutritional quality of the products promoted by these characters has decreased. [141]

In 2006, a Joint Task Force on Media and Childhood Obesity was established to examine the impact of media on childhood obesity and to develop voluntary industry standards to limit advertising that targets children. Senators Sam Brownback and Tom Harkin, former Federal Communications Commission (FCC) Chairman Kevin Martin, and former FCC Commissioner Deborah Taylor Tate convened the Task Force and members spanned from industry to government, and many others. The Task Force was unable to agree on either a uniform set of nutritional standards for defining healthy versus unhealthy foods, or media companies' obligations to enforce advertising limits.

That same year, the Council of Better Business Bureaus established the Children's Food and Beverage Advertising Initiative (CFBAI) in response to growing public concern and calls for the food and beverage industry to self-regulate. CFBAI was intended to change the ratio of food and beverage advertising messages directed to children under the age of 12 to encourage healthier eating and lifestyles.[142] Its 16 current member companies (Burger King, Cadbury Adams, Campbell Soup, Coca-Cola, ConAgra Foods, Dannon, General Mills, Hershey, Kellogg, Kraft, Mars, McDonald's, Nestle, PepsiCo, Post Foods, and Unilever) have agreed upon five central components:

1. 100% of child-directed television, print, radio, and internet advertising must promote "healthier dietary choices" or "better-for-you" products;[143]
2. Products depicted in child-directed interactive games must be "better-for-you" foods or the games must incorporate healthy lifestyle messages;
3. Companies must reduce their use of third-party licensed characters in advertising that does not promote healthy dietary choices or healthy lifestyles;
4. Companies must not pay for or actively seek placement of their products in entertainment directed at children; and
5. Companies must not advertise food or beverage products in elementary schools.

Since its implementation, the efficacy of the CFBAI's efforts has been subject to debate. FTC's 2008 report noted that the participating companies' nutritional standards, as well as their definitions of "child-directed," vary by company.[144] Within certain guidelines, each company developed its own nutritional standards for what constitutes a "better for you" food or a "healthy dietary choice." Moreover, the FTC criticized the program for applying these standards only to certain forms of advertising. It recommended, among other things, that the CFBAI improve the quality and consistency of the nutritional standards and extend those standards to all advertising and promotional techniques, including product packaging and "point-of-sale" advertising (such as displays near a check-out counter).[145]

A recent study analyzed the effectiveness of the CFBAI and found that it had not substantially shifted advertising for children toward healthier products.[146] Using one measure of nutritional quality, the study determined that, in 2009, advertisements for healthy products accounted for a very small fraction of all advertising by participating companies, while most advertising promoted foods of low nutritional value.[147] The study also found that companies participating in the CFBAI nearly doubled the use of licensed characters over the past four years, increasing from use in 8.8% of advertisements in 2005 to 15.2% in 2009. Roughly half of all advertisements with these characters are for foods in the lowest nutritional category.[148] The CFBAI has criticized this study, and argues that its voluntary efforts have led to significant improvements in foods advertised to children.[149]

Some media and entertainment companies have adopted policies limiting the types of foods for which they will license their popular characters.[150] In addition, one company has set nutritional standards for the food advertising it accepts on child-directed programming.[151] However, not all companies with popular entertainment properties have instituted similar policies, and the ones that have often use varying guidelines.

Concern about the ineffectiveness of industry self-regulation led Congress in 2009 to direct the formation of an Interagency Working Group on Food Marketed to Children (IWG).[152] This group, comprised of representatives of the FTC, FDA, CDC, and USDA, was tasked with developing recommendations for uniform standards for foods marketed to children ages 17 and under, as well as the scope of media to which such standards should apply. The group released tentative voluntary standards in December 2009 and is expected to publish proposed standards in the Federal Register for public comment in the near future.

An examination of the food and beverage industry's efforts to voluntarily limit marketing to children suggests the following conditions are necessary for meaningful improvement to occur through industry-directed initiatives:

1. First, self-regulatory groups must adopt a uniform set of nutritional standards. Without clear, consistent standards, there can be no objective basis for comparing different food products or measuring progress. The freedom of the CFBAI members to define what constitutes a "betterfor-you" food product has resulted in variations in the nutritional criteria used from one company to the next.[153] The IWG's forthcoming recommendations on standards should be helpful here More generally, Federal agencies with expertise in this area should work with industry to establish consistent standards based on the *Dietary Guidelines* that can be easily understood by both consumers and industry.
2. Second, any framework for voluntary reform must provide a level competitive playing field within the industry. If compliance results in significant competitive disadvantages to participating companies, long-term compliance becomes unsustainable. It is therefore critical to have broad participation by all companies that market food and beverage products to children. These efforts must be supported by cooperation from the major media companies that target child audiences. Media companies can directly control the type and volume of advertisements shown on their platforms. Accordingly, they can impose limits on advertising, regardless of advertisers' participation in a voluntary scheme. Media companies' use of uniform nutritional criteria would facilitate these efforts.
3. Third, to create a meaningful impact, self-regulation must apply to all forms of marketing across multiple platforms. The current voluntary guidelines allow extensive marketing of non- nutritious foods in a myriad of ways that target children.
4. Finally, effective voluntary reform will only occur if companies are presented with sufficient reasons to comply. The prospect of regulation or legislation has often served as a catalyst for driving meaningful reform in other industries and may do so in the context of food marketing as well.

The Role of Federal Regulation of Advertising

The Federal Communications Commission (FCC)'s regulatory authority varies across industries and platforms. The FCC has some direct authority to regulate advertising on children's television programs. The Children's Television Act limits the amount of commercial matter aired during children's programming to no more than 10.5 minutes per hour on weekends and no more than 12 minutes per hour on weekdays. As implemented by the FCC, these limits apply to commercial television licensees, cable operators, and satellite television (DBS) providers. In addition, the Act specifically authorizes the FCC to review and evaluate the advertising duration limitations, and to modify them in accordance with the public interest based on demonstrated need.[154]

The FTC, which has extensively studied food marketing to children,[155] is responsible for protecting consumers by preventing unfair or deceptive advertising. However, its ability to regulate child-directed advertising is limited. In 1981, in response to the FTC's effort to regulate the advertising of sugary foods to children, Congress prohibited the agency from using its authority over unfair practices to adopt rules regarding children's food advertising.

While new or revised rules to limit advertising during children's programming may be helpful or even necessary to fully address the childhood obesity epidemic, such efforts must carefully consider freedom of speech interests. Furthermore, even if efforts to limit marketing to children are successful, they would only provide a partial solution given that children are heavily exposed to advertising not specifically directed to them. For example, half of the food advertisements children see on television occur on prime-time and other non-child directed programs.[156] Programs like *American Idol* and *The Simpsons*, which are popular among children and teens, are regarded as general audience or family programming because adults form such a large share of the audience.[157] In addition, children are increasingly exposed to many forms of marketing other than television advertising, including billboards, point-of-purchase displays, and content accessed through the Internet, mobile phones, and MP3 players.

Recommendations

The Federal government can play a crucial role in improving the media environment for children with respect to the marketing of foods and beverages. It can do so while fully respecting the First Amendment right to free speech Generally, this role includes:

- Bringing together key stakeholders to develop collaborative solutions;
- Providing guidance to industry on voluntary initiatives;
- Conducting consumer education and outreach campaigns; and
- Promulgating laws and regulations when other methods prove insufficient.

Recommendation 2.5: The food and beverage industry should extend its self-regulatory program to cover all forms of marketing to children, and food retailers should avoid in-store marketing that promotes unhealthy products to children. Currently, the CFBAI guidelines limit only certain types of child-directed advertising—including television, print, radio, and Internet—but do not apply to in-store advertising, product packaging, and many other forms of marketing. For truly meaningful and effective self-regulation, all forms of child-directed marketing should be covered. Retailers have an important role to play in this effort as well, since they control what products are placed at children's eye level and can impact in-store advertising, including at the point-of-sale.

Recommendation 2.6: All media and entertainment companies should limit the licensing of their popular characters to food and beverage products that are healthy and consistent with science- based nutrition standards.

Recommendation 2.7: The food and beverage industry and the media and entertainment industry should jointly adopt meaningful, uniform nutrition standards for marketing food and beverages to children, as well as a uniform standard for what constitutes marketing to children. All nutrition standards should be based on the Dietary Guidelines. As part of this effort, the food and beverage industry should develop aggressive targets and metrics for increasing the proportion of advertisements for healthy foods and beverages across all marketing channels and platforms. The media and entertainment industry should develop uniform guidelines to ensure that a higher proportion of advertisements shown on their networks and platforms are for healthy foods and beverages.

Recommendation 2.8: Industry should provide technology to help consumers distinguish between advertisements for healthy and unhealthy foods and to limit their children's exposure to unhealthy food advertisements. The food and beverage industry and the media and entertainment industry should create an on-air labeling system that helps consumers easily distinguish between advertising for healthy and unhealthy foods. The FCC could also urge these industries to create innovative technologies that allow parents to block unhealthy food and beverage advertising from all programming. The nutritional standards should be uniform and based on the Dietary Guidelines.

Recommendation 2.9: If voluntary efforts to limit the marketing of less healthy foods and beverages to children do not yield substantial results, the FCC could consider revisiting and modernizing rules on commercial time during children's programming.

Benchmarks of Success

A substantial yearly increase in the proportion of healthy food and beverage advertisements targeting children such that, within three years, the majority of food and beverage advertisements directed to children promote healthy foods.

A substantial yearly decrease in the use of licensed characters to promote foods and beverages that are not healthy such that, within three years, licensed characters are used only to promote healthy foods and beverages.

To measure progress, data-driven studies are needed to evaluate the nutritional content of foods advertised to children. The FTC's follow up study, expected in 2011, will explore this issue, as well as shifts in consumption that have occurred following the implementation of industry self-regulation. It is critical to monitor and evaluate progress to support marketing efforts that reduce childhood obesity. If industries and government begin implementing recommendations immediately, meaningful progress could be achieved in three years.

C. Health Care Services

BMI Measurement and Obesity Prevention

Parents and caregivers often do not realize when a child is overweight or obese. In fact, studies have consistently shown that parents do not accurately perceive the weight of their overweight or obese child.[158] To inform and make potentially serious health issues salient to parents and caregivers, several states and municipalities now require children's BMI to be measured and shared with parents or caregivers. When aggregated, this data can also show the weight status over time in a student population, monitor progress of national health objectives,[159] and monitor the effects of school-based physical activity and nutrition policies and programs.

BMI is a measure of weight status at one point in time, so it is important for students, families, and policy-makers to respond to trends in BMI measurements rather than one measurement point. For children and teenagers, BMI is used as a screening tool, not a diagnostic tool, meaning that it can suggest a child has a weight concern but does not determine a child's weight status.[160] To understand a BMI score more accurately, health care providers often look at other measures. Additional assessments and tests can include a patient's medical history, family history, diet, physical activity habits, and blood pressure, and laboratory tests such as cholesterol levels. By performing follow up assessments and tests, practitioners can determine if the student actually has excess body fat or other health risks related to obesity.

A recent survey of practicing pediatricians found that nearly all respondents reported measuring height and weight at well-child visits, using growth charts as a reference. However, only about half calculate and assess BMI percentile for gender and age for children older than two years of age.[161] Most pediatricians reported that they lacked time to counsel on overweight or obesity and counseling alone has poor results, yet they noted that having simple diet and exercise recommendations would be helpful. In another survey, only about 37% of overweight children and adolescents reported being told by a health care provider they were overweight.[162]

Some states are implementing school-based BMI measurement programs. These screening programs are designed to assess the weight status of individual students to detect those who are at risk for weight-related health problems. Screening results are sent to parents and typically include: the child's BMI-for-age percentile; an explanation of the results; recommended follow up actions, if any; and tips on healthy eating, physical activity, and healthy weight management. To date, few studies have assessed the utility of these programs in preventing increases in obesity or their impact on weight-related knowledge, attitudes, and the behaviors of young people and their families.[163] These approaches merit further evaluation and review.

It is critical that health providers engage in BMI measurement. As the Surgeon General has noted, "people access the health care system through multiple channels, and medical care settings are an important avenue for preventing and controlling overweight and obesity. Clinicians are often the most trusted source of health information and can be powerful role models for healthy lifestyle habits."[164] While uninsured families have decreased access to well-child care and thus BMI screening, the recently-enacted Affordable Care Act will expand health care coverage and provide additional opportunities to support children's health.

Parents and families should also receive specific information and counseling on healthy behaviors from their health care providers. These behaviors include increasing fruit and vegetable intake and physical activity time, limiting unhealthy behaviors such as consumption of high calorie foods with little nutritional value and sugar sweetened beverage intake, and reducing sedentary time. Providers should also be able to refer parents and caregivers to the appropriate community resources.

An expert committee, convened by the American Medical Association (AMA), HHS's Health Resources and Services Administration (HRSA), and the CDC, made recommendations, which have been endorsed by the American Academy of Pediatrics (AAP), on the prevention, assessment, and treatment of children who are overweight or obese.[165] The committee noted that health care provider offices and health care systems may need to change their organizational approach to effectively address obesity prevention. More comprehensive and more useful care can be provided by integrating community resources, health care, and patient and family self-management. Health care providers may also need training on how to raise these issues most effectively with parents, since the stigma often associated with obesity can sometimes prevent clinicians from feeling comfortable discussing the implications of a high BMI.[166] Similarly, it is important to avoid children feeling stigmatized due to their weight.[167]

Obesity Treatment

The AAP-endorsed recommendations of the expert committee described above include four stages of treating obesity. The first stage is brief counseling, which can be delivered in a health care office. Subsequent stages require more time and resources. Stage two is a structured plan, consisting of a balanced diet, supervised physical activity, reduced screen time, and logs to monitor behavior change. Stages three and four include intensive interventions administered by expert obesity management professionals.[168]

The chronic care model also creates a new structure for treatment of chronic diseases by integrating community resources with health care and patient self-management. This approach is recommended for children who are overweight or obese.[169] The United States Preventive Services Task Force (USPSTF) found that effective, comprehensive weight-management programs for obese children ages 6 years and older incorporated counseling and other interventions that targeted diet and physical activity. Interventions also included behavioral management techniques to assist behavior change, and those that focused on younger children incorporated parental involvement.[170]

Recommendations

Recommendation 2.10: Pediatricians should be encouraged to routinely calculate children's BMI and provide information to parents about how to help their children achieve a healthy weight. As part of the First Lady's Let's Move Initiative, the AAP pledged in February 2010 to engage in a range of efforts to achieve two primary goals:

- Calculate BMI for every child at every well-child visit beginning at age 2, and provide information to parents about how to help their child achieve a healthy weight.
- Provide "prescriptions" for healthy active living, including good nutrition and physical activity, at every well-child visit, along with information for families about the impact of healthy eating habits and regular physical activity on overall health. Pediatricians can use their own prescription pads or existing handouts, or they can opt to use the healthy active living prescriptions created by the AAP and available at www aap org/obesity/whitehouse .

Recommendation 2.11: Federally-funded and private insurance plans should cover services necessary to prevent, assess, and provide care to overweight and obese children. HHS's Center for Medicare and Medicaid Services is planning to send a letter to State Medicaid directors to clarify how these services are currently covered in Medicaid and the Children's Health Insurance Program. The recently-enacted Affordable Care Act also requires each State to design a public awareness campaign on preventive and obesity-related services available to Medicaid enrollees.[171] Starting this year, the Act also requires new private plans to cover preventive services at no charge by exempting these benefits from deductibles and other cost-sharing requirements.[172] The Indian Health Service covers these services and has proposed an initiative on early identification and treatment of childhood and adult obesity in primary care in the President's FY2011 Budget.

Recommendation 2.12: Dentists and other oral health care providers should be encouraged to promote healthy habits and counsel families on childhood obesity prevention as part of routine preventive dental care.

Recommendation 2.13: Medical and other health professional schools, health professional associations, and health care systems should ensure that health care providers have the necessary training and education to effectively prevent, diagnose, and treat obese and overweight children.

Benchmarks of Success

All primary care physicians should be assessing BMI at all well-child and adolescent visits by 2012.

All parents and caregivers should routinely receive nutrition and physical activity counseling from their children's health care providers by 2012.

BMI assessment and counseling trends can be tracked using the National Ambulatory Medical Care Survey. Additionally, in 2009 the National Committee on Quality Assurance (NCQA) added rates of BMI assessment and nutrition and physical activity counseling for children and adolescents to its "HEDIS" (Healthcare Effectiveness Data and Information Set) quality measures. The NCQA HEDIS measures provide a complementary tool for future tracking of provider assessment and counseling trends.

Key Questions for Future Research

Building the science for prevention will help to strengthen childhood obesity prevention efforts. Below are identified research areas for consideration when developing national research agendas:

- Research the link between traditional as well as non-television forms of advertising, such as the internet, and food preferences and consumption by children and adolescents.
- Test studies of family-based interventions (such as studies of parenting style, home availability of healthful food, and opportunities for physical activity).
- Identify and test approaches for community partnerships to disseminate and implement evidence-based obesity prevention programs.
- Understand how individuals interpret and are influenced by dietary and physical activity messages (such as interpersonal, cultural, and media messages, as well as food labels) through research on learning, cognition, information processing, persuasive communications, and message framing.

- Determine whether federal farm promotion ("check-off") programs that promote certain agricultural products have an impact on Americans' compliance with the *Dietary Guidelines*.
- Compare medical and surgical treatments and lifestyle changes to identify those that are most effective in improving obesity and health outcomes in children and adolescents.
- Test models for delivering obesity prevention and treatment to change the behaviors of health practitioners and translate or disseminate evidenced-based therapies to primary care practices.
- Examine effects of targeted strategies focused on subpopulations at elevated obesity risk, such as those in racial and ethnic minority populations, tribal populations, lower socioeconomic status, rural communities, people with disabilities, and individuals taking medications that can increase body weight (such as psychotropics or insulin).
- Examine the efficacy of increased habitual sleep time on metabolic regulation such as reducing body weight, regulating appetite, and improving glucose tolerance and insulin sensitivity.

III. Healthy Food in Schools

The school environment strongly impacts the behavior, and thus the health and well-being of the students. Over 55 million American children are enrolled in elementary or secondary school.[173] These children spend over six hours each day at school, on average.[174] Over 90% of enrollees attend schools that offer one or more Federal nutrition assistance programs.[175] In addition, many students consume foods sold at school, but outside the school meal programs. Most children eat at least one meal at school, either brought from home or provided by the school. Many will have more than one meal, along with snacks and other supplementary foods.

Beyond this, various educational and related activities, both at school and traveling to and from school, have an important impact on students' nutrition and physical activity behaviors. Children's choices depend on what is most visible and easily accessible; seemingly small differences in the school environment can have large effects on what children eat. The "choice architecture" intentionally or unintentionally designed into the school nutrition environment can make a decisive difference in our children's behaviors and health.

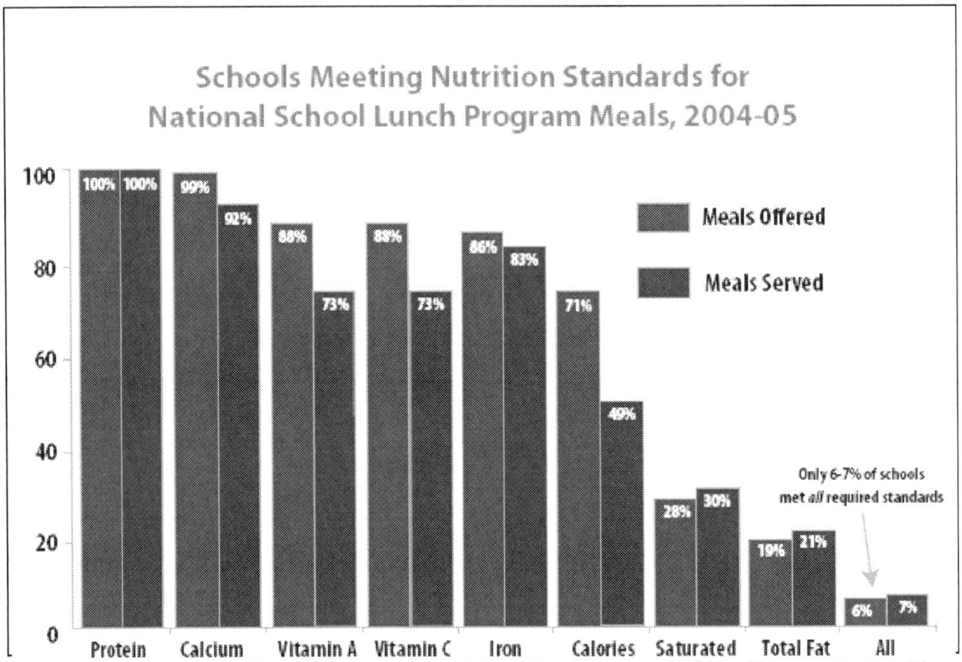

Source: U.S. Department of Agriculture, Food and Nutrition Service, Office of Research, Nutrition and Analysis, School Nutrition Dietary Assessment Study-III, Vol. I: School Foodservice, School Food Environment, and Meals Offered and Served, by Anne Gordon, et al. Project Officer: Patricia McKinney. Alexandria, VA: 2007

Unfortunately, some key aspects of current school meals, other foods at school, and environmental factors are contributing to obesity and failing to support good nutrition and physical activity behaviors. This chapter outlines a range of actions that families, communities, businesses, and governments at all levels can take to improve school foods and the school nutrition environment so they support and foster healthier food choices and help reduce childhood obesity. It focuses on four major areas:

- improvements in the quality of school meals;
- changes in other foods available at school to ensure that all food sold at school support healthful diets;
- modifications to curriculum, school program operations, and community policies and infrastructure to match changes in school foods; and
- revisions to policies and practices in juvenile justice and other institutional settings to ensure that all childhood and youth environments support healthy eating

A. Quality School Meals

Meals provided under the federally-financed National School Lunch Program and School Breakfast Program must meet a range of food-based and nutrient-based standards to ensure they contribute effectively to a good diet. The most recent national study of the content of such meals, however, found that they were not always meeting program standards.

- In the 2004-05 school year, although most school meals were consistent with meal pattern requirements and provided most key nutrients, 93-94% of meals failed to meet all nutritional standards, primarily due to not meeting standards for fat, saturated fat, or calories. [176]
- Most schools offered students the opportunity to select a balanced meal, but few students made the healthful choice. In about 90% of all schools nationwide, a student had opportunities to select low-fat lunch options, but in only about 20% of all schools did the average lunch actually selected by students meet the standards for fat.[177]
- Schools offered few whole grain foods in the school year 2004-05, and french fries and other similar potato products accounted for a disproportionate amount of the vegetable options on school lunch menus.
- Since the last time the Nutritional Standards and Meal Requirements for schools were set, the *Dietary Guidelines* have been updated. The Institute of Medicine recently provided recommendations for updated nutrition standards consistent with the 2005 Dietary Guidelines.[178] Those recommendations include increasing the amounts of fruits, vegetables and whole grains; reducing the amount of sodium and saturated fat provided; and setting a minimum and maximum number of calories for school meals. This must be done in a manner that is appealing and appetizing to children and in conjunction with effective nutrition education that helps students select and consume these foods. USDA is currently developing a regulatory proposal to guide schools in implementing updated standards.

Engaging the Community to Improve School Food: AptosMiddle School, San Francisco, CA

Beginning in the 2003-04 school year, the San Francisco Unified School District began implementing new school policies that set nutritional requirements for all foods sold in school. The changes were developed through the involvement of parents, community leaders, public health practitioners, and local physicians, spearheaded by a local organization, Parents for Public Schools in San Francisco, to implement changes in school food.

At the same time, parents at San Francisco's Aptos Middle School launched an effort specific to their school to change and improve the items sold on the snack bar menu. Student input on menu choices was an important guide to the menu changes. The success of the changes at Aptos in the 2002–03 school year helped establish the basis for the city-wide standards the following year.

The results include:

- Increased student satisfaction with school meals and increased participation in school meals programs.
- Increased service of fruits and vegetables.
- Better nutritional content of a la carte foods and increased revenue.

Source: Wojcicki, J.M., Heyman, M B (2006). Healthier Choices and Increased Participation in a Middle School Lunch Program: Effects of Nutrition Policy Changes in San Francisco *American Journal of Public Health*, 96(9), 1542-1547

Recommendations

The meals served through the National School Lunch Program (NSLP) and the School Breakfast Program (SBP) are the main nutrition intervention in elementary and secondary schools, and are a substantial part of the diets of many school children. For schools to contribute effectively to reshaping eating behaviors, the meals offered at schools must model healthful choices and help improve healthful dietary intakes.

Because school meals programs operate as partnerships between local schools, communities, state educational agencies, and the Federal government, a multi-faceted strategy is needed to promote positive change. Key actions can help advance this goal.

Recommendation 3.1: Update Federal nutritional standards for school meals and improve the nutritional quality of USDA commodities provided to schools. USDA should issue revised meal pattern requirements for the National School Lunch and School Breakfast Programs based on the Institute of Medicine's recommendations for standards that conform to the 2005 Dietary Guidelines for Americans. While most of the foods used to prepare program meals are purchased by schools, foods that USDA distributes to schools are an important component of school meals. In recent years, USDA has made great improvements in the nutritional profile of foods that it gives to schools through its commodity support programs by reducing fat, sodium, and added sugars in many of its offerings. USDA should continue to seek and implement more improvements from commodity suppliers and reprocessors, and ensure that ordering and distribution systems favor school foods that meet the updated standards.

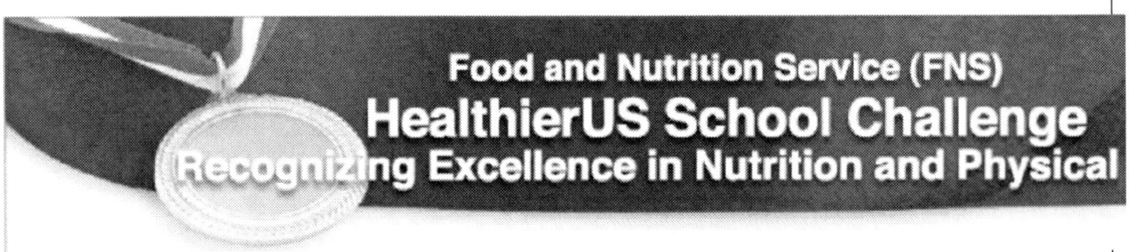

The HealthierUS Schools Challenge establishes rigorous criteria for schools' food quality, participation in meal programs, physical activity, physical education, and nutrition education–the key components that make for healthy and active kids–and provides recognition for schools that meet these criteria.

Schools can participate in this model program by going to http://www.fns.usda.gov/tn/healthierus/index. html and learning about the range of educational and technical assistance materials that promote key aspects of the Dietary Guidelines, including a Menu Planner for Healthy School Meals, which provides tips on serving more whole grains, fruits, and vegetables, and lower amounts of sugar, sodium, and saturated and trans-fats in school menus.

Food service workers in more than 75% of America's schools—along with principals, superintendents, and school board members across America—have committed to work together to reach Let's Move! Challenge goals.

Recommendation 3.2: Increase resources for school meals. Improving meals requires an investment in better foods, as well as modernized preparation and service equipment. Costs for meal programs are shared by Federal, Tribal and state governments and families of participating children, and they each have a role in supporting meal improvements.

- The Federal government should increase program reimbursements to support the provision of healthier foods.
- States and local communities should ensure that only costs that support preparation and service of school meals are charged to food service accounts, and seek opportunities to focus additional resources on meal improvements as budgets permit.
- Local communities should review their school meal pricing policies to ensure that revenue for meals only partially subsidized by USDA (i.e. "paid meals") keeps pace with free meals, in order to support full and prompt implementation of updated meals.
- School food service companies and other suppliers should constantly seek ways to improve the nutritional quality of the food they provide without increasing prices.

Recommendation 3.3: USDA should continue its outreach and technical assistance to help provide training for school food service professionals. To provide top-quality meals that are both healthy and appealing to students, local food service professionals need the tools, skills, and techniques to prepare and serve those meals. USDA should continue its program to build skills through guidance and technical assistance, and develop updated resources to support new standards School districts should be encouraged to make meal improvements, as well as the food preparation training and knowledge a priority for their local food service team. Tribal, state and local policymakers can support these changes with accreditation requirements for food service professionals, and training funds to meet and sustain the requirements. Private sector partners, from philanthropy to chefs, can help support and provide this training.

Recommendation 3.4: Schools should consider upgrading their cafeteria equipment to support the provision of healthier foods, for example, by swapping out deep fryers for salad bars. Federal resources that were recently made available for this purpose were heavily over-subscribed, indicating a strong level of local interest in making these kinds of changes. To supplement public resources, private companies that manufacture this equipment, companies that benefit from the sales of healthier products, and philanthropic partners should explore ways to make these items more affordable for schools.

Recommendation 3.5: USDA should work with all stakeholders to develop innovative ways to encourage students to make healthier choices. Putting better meals on the lunch line is not enough. The prominence, visibility, and easy accessibility of particular foods greatly matter and will inevitably have an effect on choice.[179] Where possible, healthy foods should be offered and presented in ways that encourage students to choose and consume them. This can improve students' food selection and consumption. For example, schools can automatically provide vegetables with an entrée unless the student switches to a less nutritious side dish. USDA should support the development and demonstration of innovative strategies and schools should use them to make healthy meal choices easy and compelling for students.

Recommendation 3.6: USDA should work to connect school meals programs to local growers, and use farm-to-school programs, where possible, to incorporate more fresh, appealing food in school meals. Schools should be encouraged to seek opportunities to purchase foods from local farm cooperatives. USDA should work through its "Know Your Farmer, Know Your Food" initiative and Farm to School Tactical Team to identify and eliminate regulatory barriers to local procurement, assist schools in accessing local markets, and enable food producers to effectively serve their local schools. USDA, the Bureau of Indian Affairs and the Bureau of Indian Education at the Department of the Interior, should also collaborate to increase local, traditionally appropriate foods in Tribally-controlled school meal programs, such as bison and salmon.

LISTENING TO STUDENT CUSTOMERS:"NOTHANKYOU BITES" AT BALTIMORE PUBLIC SCHOOLS

Chef Tony Geraci, Baltimore City Food Service Director, has undertaken a wide variety of strategies to engage students in making healthier choices in his low-income district. One of the most innovative is "No Thank You Bites," in which schools make available to students two-ounce samples of a new entrée, fruit or vegetable item. Students that try a sample are given star stickers. Each month, students with stars are invited to a "Constellation Party," at which Geraci and other district food service professionals are able to talk to the students about their preferences among the samples, and meal offerings more generally. Samples that are popular become part of the menu, and all of the input is used to shape future options.

As Geraci explained in Congressional testimony last fall, "We're treating kids like the savvy consumers they are.... If a student likes what she tries, great. If not, she simply says, 'No thank you. ' But everyone who works with us to expand their palates and their minds is rewarded and we listen to their suggestions. "

Recommendation 3.7: Schools should be encouraged to make improvements in their school meal programs through the HealthierUS Schools Challenge in advance of updated Federal standards. While Federal school meal standards are being updated, schools should be encouraged to start immediately

to improve their food offerings by committing to meeting the Challenge. Many already have, with over 650 schools certified to date. Challenge schools meet a range of high standards for the quality of school meals and all food sold in school, as well as a number of other important criteria. As part of the First Lady's Let's Move campaign, the Administration is actively promoting and encouraging schools to meet the Challenge criteria. Food service workers in more than 75% of America's schools—along with principals, superintendents, and school board members across America—have already committed to work together on this effort. [180]

Benchmarks of Success

Achieving the HealthierUS School Challenge goals. Double the number of schools that meet the Challenge criteria by June 2011, and add another thousand schools in each of the following two years.

All elementary and secondary schools offering meal options that meet standards for total fat and saturated fat by 2015. This can be measured by the USDA-commissioned School Nutrition Dietary Assessment Study. Assuming funds continue to be made available for this survey on a regular five year schedule, data on school year 2014-15 would be published in early 2017.

B. Other Foods in Schools

Foods offered in addition to and in competition with the meal program often do not contribute to a good diet. Such foods can be sold in the cafeteria, snack bars, vending machines, or other venues. Unlike foods served as part of the school meals programs, these foods are exempt from most Federal nutrition requirements. Often prominent and visible in schools, they contribute to obesity and unhealthy food choices.

A la carte lines allow students to choose cafeteria foods that may be part of a Federally-reimbursable program meal, without choosing healthy meal components that make that meal consistent with nutrition

standards. As a result, students who choose a la carte foods are less likely to consume appropriate amounts of key foods and nutrients than those who do not. [181]

Many schools offer foods in vending and snack bars that may undermine more balanced offerings at meal time. Foods commonly available in these venues include cookies, crackers, pastries, and other high-fat baked goods, as well as salty snacks and sports drinks. [182]

Some schools rely on food sales to cover the cost of extracurricular activities and other expenses.[183] This can lead to offerings driven by popularity and revenue potential, rather than nutrition. However, many schools found that offering healthier foods did not decrease revenue, and in some cases, increased revenue. [184]

In too many schools, such foods facilitate poor nutritional choices for students,[185] and accustom children to poor dietary practices that may ultimately contribute to obesity. They also undermine parents' efforts to promote a healthy diet for their children. Evidence in some states reveals that setting standards for foods competing with program meals can improve students' consumption of more healthy food options.[186]

Recommendations

Like school meals, local schools must work hand-in-hand with Federal, Tribal, and state governments to reshape their competitive food policies. Key actions can help advance this goal.

Recommendation 3.8: Increase the alignment of foods sold at school, including in the a la carte lines and vending machines, with the Dietary Guidelines. Under current law, USDA has very limited authority to set and enforce standards for foods regularly sold outside the Federally-supported school meals programs. In the upcoming reauthorization of the Child Nutrition programs, the Administration is committed to gaining authority to develop and issue these standards for schools participating in USDA programs, and the food and beverage industry has stated its strong support for Congress providing USDA with this authority. [187] The standards would be developed through a transparent and participatory public rulemaking process, and the Institute of Medicine's evidence-based recommendations for such standards[188] can serve as a foundation for the USDA's proposal.

Recommendation 3.9: Food companies should be encouraged to develop new products and reformulate existing products so they meet nutritional standards based on the Dietary Guidelines and appeal to children. Food manufacturers and marketers have a critical role to play in meeting new standards, and have already shown an ability to adapt their products to appeal to more nutrition-conscious consumers over the past several years. These industries should be encouraged to continue to use their energy and ingenuity to develop foods that schools can offer within and outside of the school meals programs. These foods should support healthy diets and offer the taste and convenience needed to appeal to students For example, food companies should be encouraged to:

- Offer whole grain-rich bread and cereal products such as sandwich rolls and pastas;
- Reformulate entrees, sauces, and condiments to contain less sodium, while incorporating alternative flavorings and seasonings to maintain palatability; and
- Reduce the high levels of added sugars in many flavored milks and yogurts.

Benchmarks of Success

Assuming new Federal standards for the nutritional quality of all foods in schools are in effect by 2013, schools should achieve full substantive compliance by that date. In the meantime, progress can be measured by an increase in the number of schools meeting the HealthierUS School Challenge, described above "Substantive compliance" is meant to denote full consistency between all foods sold in school and Federal standards; any non-compliant schools should be working on USDA-approved corrective actions to achieve substantive compliance.

C. Food-Related Factors in the School Environment

Many facets of the school setting can affect children's dietary choices. Some operate directly on their eating behaviors, while others are more subtle. In too many schools, the connection between service of meals and other foods at school and the responsibility to educate, enable, and motivate healthful nutrition habits is weak or non-existent.

Nutrition Education

More, and better, nutrition education is needed in many schools. While approximately 75% of schools require nutrition education as part of health curriculum requirements, the time spent on nutrition and dietary behavior has declined in recent years, and funding has been limited.[189] Many teachers are not equipped with the skills and knowledge to integrate and promote nutrition education into their classroom curricula. Research has shown that nutrition education interventions, if well designed and effectively implemented can improve dietary behaviors.[190]

Lunch Room Environment

Eating behaviors can also be shaped by the cafeteria and lunch room setting, such as the display and description of food and beverages, pricing and methods of payment, and the length of time and time of day made available to eat.[191] Some experiments indicate that these factors can promote healthy choices,[192] although it is not yet clear precisely how such strategies can best be applied in schools.

In addition, some schools' meal service arrangements discourage some children, particularly low-income children, from taking advantage of school meals, undermining the impact of improvements in the nutritional quality of those meals. For example, one survey found that one-third of high schools had separate lines or rooms for the school lunch program and competitive foods In many of those schools, the vast majority of the students standing in the lunch line were low income.[193] Marketing of food and beverages within schools has also grown substantially in recent years, and may influence food choices in ways that do not contribute to good health.[194]

In addition, some middle and high schools permit students to leave campus for lunch. One study found that 29% of high schools reported having an "open campus" lunch policy.[195] For those who eat lunch off-campus, improvements in school meals will have little impact on their dietary intake. Some schools are also surrounded by fast-food restaurants with few healthy options.[196]

Schools should also be made aware of factors that can impact a child's decision about what to eat, including food allergies and religious restrictions, and they should be encouraged to use existing options to accommodate children's needs.

Recommendations

Recommendation 3.10: USDA and the U.S. Department of Education should collaborate with states to increase the availability and consistency of nutrition education in schools. States should be encouraged to ensure that teacher preparation requirements include basic nutrition knowledge and nutrition education as part of every teacher's skill set. USDA and the U.S. Department of Education should work together to improve national standards and requirements for nutrition education. Teachers in local schools can explore interdisciplinary approaches to incorporate healthy eating in the school curriculum (for example, history may have a subject related to healthy diets, math may include how to calculate the needed caloric intake, foreign languages may have students design a menu). The Bureau of Indian Education, Teach for America, and other teacher corps programs could also expand their partnership to include nutrition education.

Recommendation 3.11: Where possible, use school gardens to educate students about healthy eating. School gardens offer opportunities for fun and physical activity while also serving as an important educational tool to help students understand how healthful food is produced. Some research suggests that school gardens used as part of a nutrition education strategy can increase knowledge of fruits and vegetables and influence behavior change among children.[197] Schools can further make the link between agriculture and nutritious food by inviting local farmers markets to operate from area school yards. Parents and students can also share their knowledge when shopping together for locally grown fruits and vegetables or participating in Community Supported Agriculture programs.

Recommendation 3.12: Technical assistance should be provided to schools about how to a cafeteria and lunch room environment can support and encourage a healthful meal. Factors such as the timing and length of the meal period; cleanliness and noise level in the dining room; and adequate space for eating can all play a role in what children consume.

Recommendation 3.13: Schools should be encouraged to ensure that choosing a healthy school meal does not have a social cost for a child. Efforts that make school meals more nutritious and appealing cannot effectively improve students' choices if other factors undermine their opportunity to select them. For example, many schools provide reimbursable meals at a different serving station than a la carte foods Children can be discouraged from considering full meals if they are not exposed to them. Furthermore, in schools where most meals are served free or at reduced-price, separating lines can create a perception that program meals are intended only for lower-income students, potentially creating a stigma that prevents children who cannot afford a la carte food from eating at all.[198] Schools should be encouraged to examine their operational practices to ensure that all students have a full opportunity to consider and choose a school meal.

Recommendation 3.14: Schools should be encouraged to consider the impact of food marketing on education. Food marketing can occur at school in a number of forms, including on scoreboards, food display cases, and vending machines; in student publications, educational materials provided "free" by food firms, branded fundraisers and food reward programs; and even market research conducted on campus.[199] Schools should be encouraged to limit school-based marketing that contributes to poor health. Private companies should be encouraged to voluntarily shift towards the promotion of healthy foods and away from advertising that promotes unhealthy products.

Recommendation 3.15: School districts should be encouraged to create, post, and implement a strong local school wellness policy. Recognizing the critical role schools play in promoting students' health, preventing childhood obesity, and combating poor nutrition and physical inactivity, Congress passed a law requiring school districts to establish a local wellness policy in 2004. This policy would sets goals for nutrition education, physical activity, campus food provision, and other school-based activities designed to promote student wellness. School boards and other community leaders should work to ensure this policy reflects the abovementioned recommendations, while tailoring them to their communities' needs. Tribes can work with the National Indian Education Association and National Indian School Board Association to develop an effective school wellness policy that reflects Tribal values and culture. USDA should also seek authority in the Child Nutrition and WIC Reauthorization Act to strengthen school wellness policy development, implementation, monitoring, and evaluation. The U S Department of Education should work with USDA to support these efforts.

To aid in the development and implementation of the wellness policy, schools should consider establishing

a health advisory council, as a number of communities have done. These councils, comprised of school officials and staff, parents, local public health authorities, and other community members, foster an exchange of information on a wide range of issues that influence the local school environment. They also provide support, oversight, and accountability for school nutrition improvement efforts.[200]

Benchmarks of Success

Increase in the number of school districts that provide a healthful school environment, which could include such features as nutrition education integrated into school programming; lunch room environments that support healthy eating; strong marketing policies; and a school health advisory council. Progress can be assessed using data from the School Health Policies and Programs Study (SHPPS), which is conducted every six years by CDC's National Center for Chronic Disease Prevention and Health Promotion. The most recent SHPPS data is for 2006; the next study will be done in 2012 and released in 2013.

D. Food in Other Institutions

Other institutions that play a significant role in the lives of children and young adults do not consistently support healthful nutrition behaviors.

Afterschool Programs

For many children, school activities do not end when the last bell rings. Afterschool programs, such as expanded day care centers, tutoring and other instruction programs, and 21st Century Community Learning Centers, serve children in elementary schools across the nation. In 2008, 56% of public elementary schools offered one or more such programs.[201] As with school during regular hours, the afterschool environment influences the eating behaviors of participating children. Because many of these programs operate in low-income communities where access to food may be more limited, incorporating healthful meals and snacks can be especially important. Federally-supported afterschool snacks are available through the National School Lunch Program (NSLP) and the Child and Adult Care Food Program (CACFP). Support for more substantial meals like supper is available through CACFP for low-income communities, but currently in only a limited number of states.

Juvenile Detention and Correctional Settings

While limited research exists on the nutritional services for youth in the juvenile detention and correctional facilities, anecdotal evidence suggests that many detained and incarcerated youth consume diets high in fat, cholesterol, and sodium and low in fresh fruit and vegetables. These types of diets are particularly problematic for incarcerated youth with special dietary needs. In addition, facilities may not employ or have access to licensed nutritionists or dietitians to oversee institutional food services.

Providing appropriate nutrition in juvenile detention and correctional settings is underscored by the population size and the risk factors for weight related problems facing these youth. Data shows that in 2007 more than 360,000 delinquency cases resulted in youth being placed in secure detention and nearly 149,000 resulted in youth being placed out of their home. [202] During a one-day count in 2008, approximately 80,000 youth were housed in 3,000 publicly and privately operated juvenile facilities, including public, private, and tribal facilities. [203]

Many of these young people are at risk for or have serious health concerns that are often undiagnosed or untreated, and they experience physical and mental health problems at rates exceeding those in the general youth population. [204] They are frequently children who have experienced severe familial dysfunction, witnessed violence, or have been victims of physical and sexual abuse. [205]

Many juvenile detention centers operate the National School Lunch Program and School Breakfast Program, but it is unclear how many such institutions offer meals that are consistent with the programs' nutritional requirements. Effective nutrition education, institutional food services, culinary arts, and recreational programming are critical components in addressing the overall health care needs of this vulnerable group.

Recommendations

Recommendation 3.16: Promote good nutrition through afterschool programs. Afterschool programs face distinct circumstances and challenges beyond those that impact children and young people during the school day. States and communities can develop standards and strategies tailored for afterschool programs by building on and integrating the afterschool snack components of USDA's Child Nutrition programs. The Federal government could develop and offer model approaches and resources to inform these efforts.

Recommendation 3.17: Promote healthy behaviors in juvenile correctional and related facilities. States and localities should be encouraged to ensure that juvenile justice facilities use nutrition programs available to them, such as USDA's school meal programs. Federal, state, and non-governmental organizations should collaborate to develop evidence-based programs and standards for health promotion and disease prevention services, including nutrition counseling, meal services, and recreational programs that meet the needs and circumstances of juvenile justice populations. Related programs such as organic fruit and vegetable gardening, farming, and culinary arts initiatives in juvenile justice facilities can potentially promote health, education, workforce development, and positive youth development.

Benchmarks of Success

As this area is explored further, it may be appropriate to develop benchmarks to track progress in improving nutritional outcomes in these settings.

Key Questions for Future Research

- How can we make healthy foods more affordable for use in schools? And more attractive to children?

- What can we learn from behavioral economics to support healthful eating in schools, and how can schools promote healthful eating over the longer term?
- What are the correlative and/or causal linkages between exposure to food marketing in schools and food consumption patterns or obesity?
- How can effective school-based nutrition education models be identified and scaled up to national implementation?
- How does participation in the afterschool snack and meal programs supported by USDA affect children's diets, opportunities for nutrition education and physical activity?
- To what extent are health promotion and disease prevention services such as nutrition counseling, improved diet, and recreational programs, provided to youth in the juvenile justice system? What evidence-based food services, nutritional education, and exercise programming can best address the needs of youth involved in juvenile justice systems?

IV. Access to Healthy, Affordable Food

Healthy options can be hard to find in too many communities. Millions of low-income Americans live in "food deserts," neighborhoods that lack convenient access to affordable and healthy food. Instead of supermarkets or grocery stores, these communities often have an abundance of fast-food restaurants and convenience stores. In addition, stores in low-income communities may stock fewer and lower quality healthy foods. When available, the cost of fresh foods in low-income areas can be high. Public transportation to supermarkets is often lacking, and long distances separate home and supermarkets in many rural communities and American Indian reservations. It is hard for residents of these areas—even those fully informed and motivated—to follow the necessary and recommended steps to maintain a healthy weight for themselves and their children. Too often, economic incentives strongly favor unhealthy eating, and accessibility, safety concerns, and convenience can also promote unhealthy outcomes.

Limited access to healthy food choices can lead to poor diets and higher levels of obesity and other diet-related diseases. In addition, limited access to affordable food choices can lead to higher levels of food insecurity, increasing the number of low- and moderate-income families without access to enough food to sustain a healthy, active life. There is a growing, though incomplete, body of research that finds an association between food insecurity and obesity, suggesting that hunger and obesity may be two sides of the same coin.

Many communities around the country have already taken steps to make healthy and affordable foods accessible to all residents because of the potential to improve diet quality and reduce obesity, as well as to create jobs, increase local investment and economic activity, and revitalize neighborhoods. This chapter recommends a comprehensive approach that builds on a promising start to mobilize public and private sector resources to make the healthy choice the easy choice for all Americans.

Specifically, this chapter lays out four key elements for ensuring access to healthy, affordable food:

- Convenient physical access to grocery stores and other retailers that sell a variety of healthy foods;
- Prices that make healthy choices affordable and attractive;
- A range of healthy products available in the marketplace; and
- Adequate resources for consumers to make healthful choices, including access to nutrition assistance programs to meet the special needs of low-income Americans.

A. Physical Access to Healthy Food

Too many Americans live in communities with limited access to supermarkets and grocery stores Nationwide, USDA estimates that 23.5 million people, including 6.5 million children, live in low-income areas that are more than a mile from a supermarket. Of the 23.5 million, just under half have incomes at or below 200% of the poverty line, and almost 1 million do not have access to a car USDA estimates that 2.3 million people live in low-income rural areas that are more than ten miles from a supermarket; and again, just under half have low incomes.[206]

Limited access to healthy foods plays a significant role in poor dietary decisions. A scarcity of healthy foods makes it more difficult for low-income residents to adhere to a nutritious diet than for their counterparts in wealthier, resource-rich neighborhoods.[207] Residents with better access to supermarkets and limited access to convenience stores tend to have healthier diets and lower levels of obesity. Although less consistent, studies do suggest that residents with limited access to fast-food restaurants have healthier diets and lower levels of obesity. [208]

Access to supermarkets, grocery stores, and specialty markets is important, in part, because they give consumers access to a variety of fruits and vegetables. Diets rich in fruits and vegetables offer a number of health benefits[209] and have been linked to a lower prevalence of obesity or reduced weight gain. [210] Most Americans, especially those with low income, consume far fewer fruits and vegetables than recommended by current dietary guidance,[211] and a lack of easy accessibility may be one reason. A number of studies suggest that better retail access corresponds with healthier eating. Residents with more access to supermarkets or a greater abundance of healthy foods in neighborhood food stores consume more fresh produce and other healthful items. Without nearby access to healthy ingredients, families have a harder time meeting recommended dietary guidelines. [212]

Some research has found significant associations between the availability of food stores and adolescent BMI. The availability of chain supermarkets was associated with lower adolescent BMI and overweight status, while the availability of convenience stores was associated with higher adolescent BMI and overweight status. [213]

Many factors contribute to an individual's overall diet, body weight, and the risk of developing diet-related diseases such as diabetes or cardiovascular disease. Individual factors can explain some but not all of the differences in the rates in which different groups experience these problems. Attention on the relationship between retail food access and obesity has increased as researchers obtain a better understanding of the factors besides individual behaviors that may lead to differences in diet and health outcomes.

Creative tools can be used to assess a community's needs. For example, Michigan's Department of Public Health has developed an online Nutrition Environment Assessment Tool (NEAT) to help communities assess the extent to which they promote and support healthy eating. [214] The U. S. Department of Defense adopted this tool for use by commanding officers and other stakeholders to make similar assessments of military communities and facilities.[215] A number of policy interventions can lead to improved access to healthy, affordable food. Communities can bring supermarkets to underserved neighborhoods, help smaller groceries or corner stores expand their stock of healthy and affordable food, and develop other retail outlets such as farmers' markets, public markets, cooperatives, farm stands, community-supported agriculture, and mobile vendors. These efforts also create jobs, bolster local economies, and revitalize neighborhoods, contributing to local economic development. A number of communities have undertaken these kinds of efforts, through projects such as Pennsylvania's Fresh Food Financing Initiative.

FAITH-BASED ORGANIZATIONS FIND CREATIVE SOLUTIONS TO "FOOD DESERTS"

There is no one-size-fits-all solution to the problem of food deserts in America. In some communities, it may be economically feasible to bring in a supermarket and sustain it over time; in others, the solution may be a mobile grocery store that comes through town once a week but provides access to healthy foods that community residents otherwise would lack.

Some of the most creative strategies have come from faith-based organizations, many of which have a long tradition of helping to meet the food needs in their communities, through food pantries and other anti-hunger efforts. Here are just a few examples:

- The Central Detroit Christian Community Development Corporation operates the **"Peaches & Greens" Produce Truck**, which travels through the streets of central Detroit like an ice cream truck, stopping to sell fruits and vegetables to area residents. The organization has also arranged for a number of corner stores to sell "Peaches & Greens" produce.
- In South Los Angeles, the First African Methodist Episcopal Church has arranged for the **open-air So Fresh Market** to operate in its parking lot. The market welcomes families to participate in free activities and live entertainment, while fresh and natural foods are sold to promote a healthy lifestyle and patrons are invited to watch as cooks present quick and easy meal demonstrations. Partnering with the market is part of a broader effort by the church to promote healthier eating among African Americans in the community.

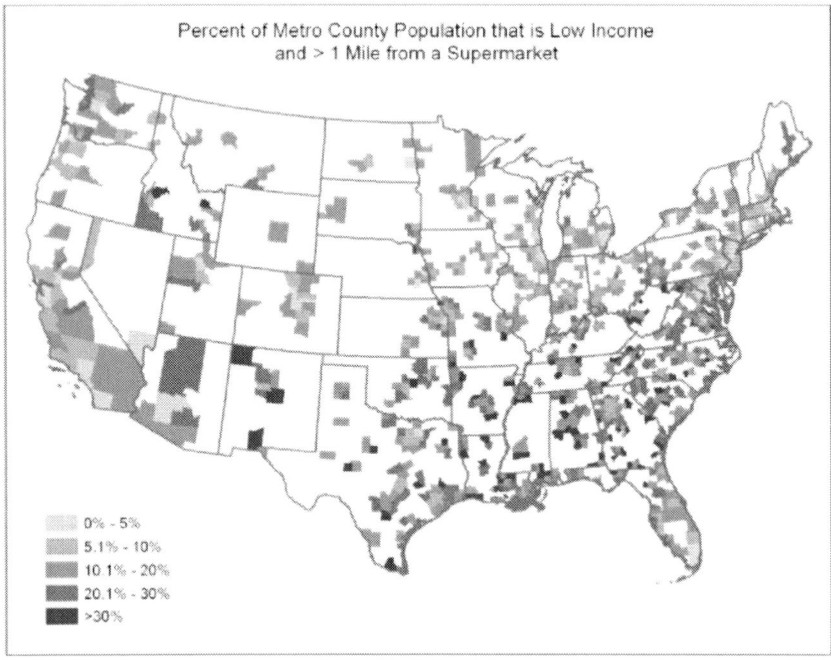

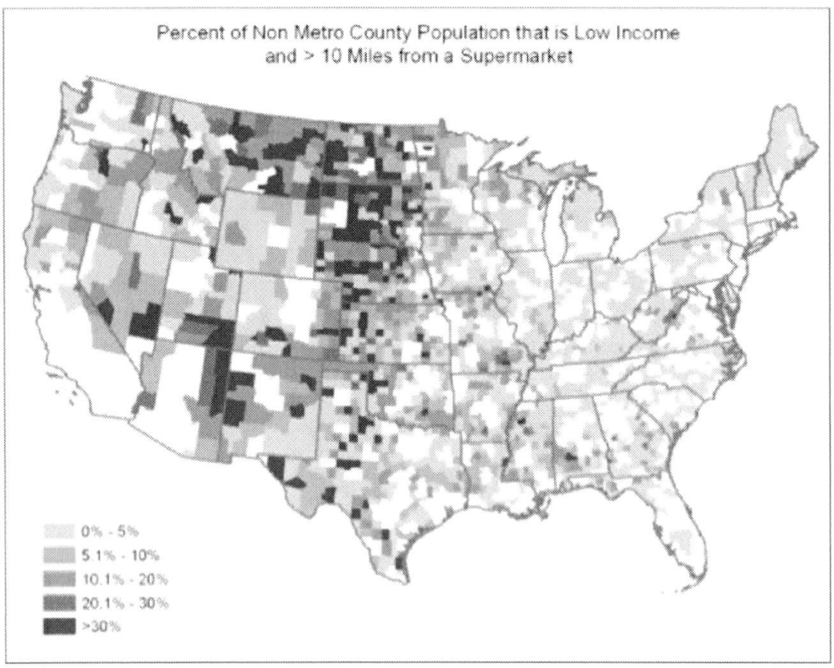

Food Deserts in Urban and Rural America.

Direct-to-consumer marketing outlets provide another path to increase healthy food access in underserved areas and stimulate economic development in rural communities across America. These opportunities, including farmers' markets, farm stands, and community supported agriculture enterprises, are currently promoted by the USDA through its Know Your Farmer, Know Your Food Initiative.

There are also many publicly and privately managed facilities that are frequented by children and their families, including at meal times, such as national, state, and local parks, as well as privately-run amusement parks, sports venues, and other recreational facilities for children. These places can be considered small scale "food deserts" because meals or snacks are available for purchase but few, if any, healthy options are available.

Recommendations

Recommendation 4.1: Launch a multi-year, multi-agency Healthy Food Financing Initiative to leverage private funds to increase the availability of affordable, healthy foods in underserved urban and rural communities across the country. As proposed in the President's FY11 Budget, through this initiative, USDA, HHS, and the Treasury Department will partner to make over $400 million available to community development financial institutions, nonprofits, public agencies and businesses to promote interventions that expand access to nutritious foods. Such interventions include helping grocery stores, small businesses, and other retailers provide healthy food options in lower-income communities. Interventions may also include helping improve supply chains to bring fruits, vegetables, and other healthy foods from rural agricultural areas to urban stores and markets. Private sector investments are a critical part of this initiative's success, since they provide up-front capital and sustain the investments until these stores have a chance to establish themselves in the community and build a strong customer base.

In addition to these new resources, communities can access existing Federal grant and loan programs, as well as state, local, and private funds to create market opportunities for producers and to support regional planning systems that ensure greater access to healthy food in underserved areas. Resources include USDA's Farmers' Market Promotion Program, Specialty Crop Block Grants, Community Food Projects, Community Facilities Program, Business and Industry Guaranteed Loan Program, Healthy Urban Food Enterprise Development Center, and Sustainable Communities Regional Planning grants; HHS' Community Economic Development Program; and the U. S. Department of Housing and Urban Development's Community Development Block Grant and Choice Neighborhood initiative.

Recommendation 4.2: Local governments should be encouraged to create incentives to attract supermarkets and grocery stores to underserved neighborhoods and improve transportation routes to healthy food retailers. Incentives could include tax credits, grant and loan programs, and small business or economic development programs. Communities could also develop zoning requirements that create safe, non-motorized routes such as sidewalks, pedestrian malls, and bicycle paths between all neighborhoods and supermarkets, grocery stores, or other retailers who sell healthy food.[216] Local communities can also commit job training resources to ensure that a well-trained workforce is available for healthy food retailers who are considering locating in their area.

LAND USE AND FOOD SYSTEM PLANNING

Many communities have had an opportunity to promote access to fresh foods and urban agriculture as a component of their land-use and food system planning processes. Across the country, projects are helping to create, enable, and fund community garden and urban agriculture programs, and developing zoning and permitting processes friendly to urban agriculture and healthy food access. Community gardens can provide culturally significant foods not available in local grocery stores. For example:

- The city of Fresno changed its zoning ordinance to allow farmers markets in all non-residential and certain single-family residential zones. Now, Fresno planners want to plan for urban agriculture in newly developing areas.
- Vendors in Kansas City who sell healthy foods pay a reduced permit fee. City planners also list recommended and excluded products for public vending in the city's parks and recreational areas.
- New York City uses a combination of incentives and restrictions to get green produce carts in areas of the city with the least access to fresh fruits and vegetables.
- Detroit and Cleveland have reclaimed acres of vacant land and lots for community gardens.

Recommendation 4.3: Food distributors should be encouraged to explore ways to use their existing distribution chains and systems to bring fresh and healthy foods into underserved communities. The private supply chains that have been developed to bring healthy foods to restaurants and less healthy items to corner stores and grocery stores should be deployed to bring healthy foods to communities that lack these retail options. USDA, as part of its Know Your Farmer, Know Your Food initiative, can also play a role in developing food hub distribution centers to increase opportunities for regional distribution.

Recommendation 4.4: Encourage communities to promote efforts to provide fruits and vegetables in a variety of settings and encourage the establishment and use of direct–to-consumer marketing outlets such as farmers' markets and community supported agriculture subscriptions. Options that communities could consider include the following:

- Promote the use of WIC cash value vouchers, WIC and Seniors Farmers' Market coupons, and SNAP benefits in farmers markets and other settings where fruits and vegetables are sold;
- Fund outreach, education, and transportation to encourage residents of lower-income neighborhoods and nutrition assistance program participants to use farmers' markets and farm stands;
- Use land use policies to promote, expand, and protect potential sites for community gardens and farmers' markets such as vacant city-owned land or unused parking lots;
- Develop community-based group activities that link procurement of affordable, healthy food with improving skills in purchasing and preparing food;
- Provide incentives to purchase and sell local native-grown produce to Indian schools and communities; and

- Consider the adoption of ordinances or by-laws that promote healthy food vendors and mobile fruit and vegetable vendors in low-income and geographically isolated neighborhoods.

Recommendation 4.5: Encourage the establishment of regional, city, or county food policy councils to enhance comprehensive food system policy that improve health. Experience in some communities has shown that food policy councils can bring together citizens and government officials to examine state or local food systems. This unique form of civic engagement assembles diverse food system stakeholders to develop food and agriculture policy recommendations.

Recommendation 4.6: Encourage publicly and privately-managed facilities that serve children, such as hospitals, afterschool programs, recreation centers, and parks (including national parks) to implement policies and practices, consistent with the Dietary Guidelines, to promote healthy foods and beverages and reduce or eliminate the availability of calorie-dense, nutrient-poor foods.

HEALTHY FOODS IN OUR PARKS

ParksHealthy food is often hard to come by on America's public lands. Traditionally, concessioners have pro-vided visitors with a limited number of options, many of which are calorie-laden and highly processed. In cafeterias and snack stands across the National Park System, concessioners are beginning to provide a broader range of healthy, organic, and local foods. The Park Service administers approximately 600 conces-sions contracts across its 392 units, grossing about $1 billion annually. Recently, individual parks have taken the lead in working with their concessioners to revamp and revitalize traditionally limited, menus.

At **Golden Gate National Parks' Muir Woods Trading Post**, Ortega Family Enterprises provides a range of low-sugar, reduced-calorie, and organic food, much of which is locally sourced. All of these items are affordably priced and have raised profits for the park and the concessioner alike. Similarly healthy offerings can be found at the company's other National Park outposts in New Mexico. Healthful concessions are also found in **Yellowstone and Grand Teton National Parks**, which offer a range of all-natural and vegetarian options. Far away from the big western parks, the Statue of Liberty boasts a range of healthy options in a densely populated urban area. **Baltimore's Fort McHenry** is preparing to open a new cafeteria based on a model school lunch program. And on the **National Mall**, concessioners are now serving low-fat snacks like fruit and yogurt and lunches like vegetable hummus wraps.

Benchmarks of Success

Eliminate food deserts in America in seven years. To monitor progress towards this goal, USDA will estimate the number of people in low income areas more than a mile from a supermarket or large grocery store (10 miles in rural areas) every three years beginning in 2012, using demographic data from the American Community Survey and store location information from commercial sources and USDA's directory of stores authorized to accept SNAP benefits.

B. Food Pricing

Prices have a large effect on consumer choices. Consumer behavior has shifted as food prices have declined and low cost, energy-dense foods have become more convenient. Technological advances have made food cheaper. One study found that food prices dropped in comparison to all other goods, over a 50 year period. [217] But these price advantages do not extend to all types of food. Over the last 30 years, prices for fruits and vegetables increased nearly twice as fast as the price of carbonated drinks. [218]

An increase in the price of fruits and vegetables relative to less healthy foods can reduce consumers' incentives to purchase fruits and vegetables, resulting in less healthy diets. Some analyses suggest that energy-dense foods composed of refined grains, added sugars, or fats remain the lowest-cost option to the consumer. [219] It is widely believed that American consumers have seen a significant increase in prices of fruits and vegetables alongside a decrease in the prices of foods that contribute to obesity. Because of quality improvements in fresh fruits and vegetables, however, it is difficult to draw conclusions about the trends in prices and incentives. One recent analysis found that prices declined for commonly consumed fresh fruits and vegetables for which quality has remained fairly constant, as well as for snack foods. This evidence suggests that the price of a healthy diet has not changed relative to an unhealthy one. [220] Nonetheless, it is not disputed that the prices of some unhealthy foods have fallen, and that prices play a significant role in consumer choices.

Prices change over time for a variety of reasons. Better production and distribution technologies generate more and better goods, driving down prices. Foods that once were available only seasonally are now available year-round. Advances in food processing and packaging have introduced a multitude of ready-to-eat foods, available virtually anywhere and anytime. Farm programs have been designed to stabilize crop prices for farmers and may affect production decisions, commodity prices, and ultimately the prices consumers pay. State and local sales taxes imposed on soft drinks, candy, and snacks raise their cost relative to other food purchases. Nutrition assistance programs subsidize meals for millions of low-income Americans, reducing the relative price of food compared to other consumer needs. As a result, there are many opportunities to affect the cost of healthy food.

Studies suggest that if the price of a particular food increases or decreases, consumption will decrease or increase. Research has found increases in purchases of healthier foods when prices are reduced, and decreases in purchases of less healthy foods as prices increase.[221] The potential influence of food prices on consumption necessitates consideration of the extent to which changes in farm, tax, and subsidy policies might affect consumption patterns.

Agriculture Policy

Since the Great Depression, American farm policy has been designed to stabilize crop prices, keep farmers producing food and fiber, and provide American families with an abundant, affordable, and reliable food supply. Eligible farmers receive support through a variety of Federal programs. Nearly all the subsidies go to growers of five commodities:

soybeans, corn, rice, wheat, and cotton. In comparison, relatively few subsidies support fruit and vegetable farmers, although the Food, Conservation, and Energy Act of 2008 included, for the first time, $1. 3 billion in new funding over 10 years for specialty crops—fruits, vegetables, and nuts—and increased programs that support local agriculture and healthy foods. It also included a pilot project to allow planting of fruits and vegetables on base acres for USDA's farm commodity price and income support programs in a limited number of states.

Additional studies should be conducted to determine whether current agricultural policy has an impact on the availability and pricing of different types of food and American diets. For example, the orientation of farm program payments toward a group of commodities may have an impact on the composition of the food supply and the relative availability of certain commodities. USDA's Economic Research Service has estimated that to establish a sufficient supply of fruits and vegetables for all Americans to meet the Dietary Guidelines, U. S. producers would have to more than double their fruit acreage (from 3.5 million acres today, to 7. 6 million) and increase vegetable acreage by nearly one and a half times (from 6.5 million acres today, to 15. 3 million). [222]

In addition, some research on the link between obesity and farm programs finds that our farm programs have had small and mixed effects on farm commodity prices, resulting in smaller effects on relative retail prices. Over the past 15 years, most farm subsidies have been in the form of direct income support that is not connected to actual production. One analysis found that direct income support did not significantly affect the affordability of food, either on the whole or within food groups.[223]

While farm subsidies have lowered some commodities' prices, their effects may be countered by policies that restrict acreage or production, which potentially increase prices. In addition, the cost of farm commodities represent only a small and shrinking share of the cost of retail food products, on average less than 19%, making changes in commodity prices translate to small changes in the prices consumers pay.[224] One study found, for example, that the corn content of high fructose corn syrup represented about 1.6% of the value of soft drink manufacturing costs and sugar just 0.1%. In turn, small changes in prices are likely to induce only small changes in consumption.[225] As noted above, however, further research can help respond to the underlying questions.

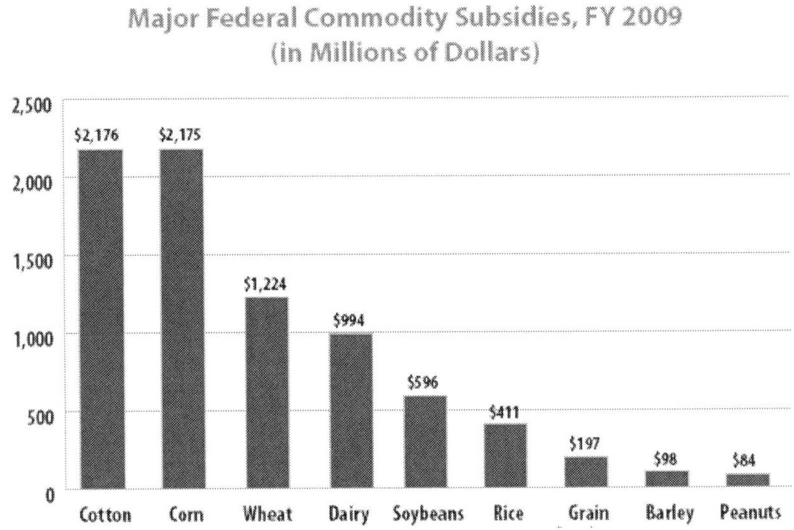

Source: U.S. Department of Agriculture. (2010). Agricultural Outlook: Statistical Indicators, Table 35. Retrieved April, 2010 from http://www.ers.usda.gov/Publications/AgOutlook/AOTables/

Retail State sales and vending machine "snack tax" rates, 2009								
	Sales Tax				Vending Machine Tax			
Product	**Number of States**	**Average Tax Rate**	**Min Rate**	**Max Rate**	**Number of States**	**Average Tax Rate**	**Min Rate**	**Max Rate**
Soda	33	5.2	1. 2	7. 0	39	5. 3	1. 2	8. 0
Candy	29	4.8	1. 0	7. 0	37	5.1	1. 0	8. 0
Gum	28	4.7	1. 0	7. 0	38	5.0	1.0	8.0
Ice cream	18	4. 2	1.0	7. 0	35	5.0	1.0	8.0
Popsicles	16	4. 0	1.0	7.0	33	5.0	1.0	8.0
Chips/pretzels	14	3.7	1.0	7.0	32	5.0	1.0	8.0
Milkshakes/ Baked goods	14	3.7	1.0	7.0	33	5.0	1.0	8.0

Source: Bridging the Gap: www impacteen org/obesitystatedata htm

Tax Policy

The Institute of Medicine and others have recommended that governments implement a tax strategy to discourage consumption of foods and beverages that have minimal nutritional value as a step in the fight against childhood obesity. Based on the notion that consumers will respond to the increased food cost by reducing their consumption, a tax could generate considerable revenue to fund obesity-fighting programs.[226] Many states already tax caloric-sweetened food and beverages.

The effectiveness of taxing food purchases primarily depends on the degree to which consumers are aware of and respond to changes in food prices. One review suggests that the percentage change in consumption is generally smaller than the percentage change in price.[227] Consumers may, however, be fairly responsive to a price change in caloric-sweetened sodas, fruit drinks, and sports drinks. The extent of the response would certainly be affected by the size of the change in price. Recent research indicates that current state-level tax rates on soda purchases have had a relatively small impact on adolescent[228] and adult weights.[229] But a higher tax rate would likely have a greater impact on consumption, as evidenced by the effects of the substantial rise in tobacco taxes.[230]

Subsidy Policy

Providing incentives or subsidies to encourage greater consumption of healthier food choices offers an alternative to taxes on foods of limited nutritional value. In experiments, targeted price changes have increased purchases of healthier snacks from vending machines. For example, a 50% price reduction on fresh fruit and baby carrots in two secondary school cafeterias resulted in a four-fold increase in fresh fruit sales and a two-fold increase in baby carrot sales.[231] Another experiment used a simple color-coded label of red (least healthy), yellow, or green (most healthy) based on fat and calorie content and added a five cent "tax" (approximately 8% of the product's value) on each red item. After one year, this resulted in a 5% decrease in sales of least healthy items, a 16% increase in the sale of most healthy items, and overall sales increased as well.[232]

A recent study on the effect of price subsidies on healthy food consumption among SNAP participants suggests that a 10% subsidy for vegetables and fruits would increase vegetable consumption from 1.26 cups to 1.33 cups per day, and fruit consumption from 0. 89 cup to 0.97 cup. These increases in consumption bring individuals closer to the recommended levels, closing the gap by 4. 7% for vegetables and 7% for fruits.[233]

Since 2005, a group of farmers markets, foundations, local governments, and nonprofit organizations have collaborated on pilot incentive programs to expand USDA programs to improve the health and nutrition of low income families and their children. Wholesome Wave's Double Value Coupon Program increases the value of SNAP and other program benefits when used at participating farmers markets, reducing the cost of fruits and vegetables for low-income participants. Initiated in 2008, the program has expanded to more than 60 markets in 12 states and the District of Columbia. Early results from participating farmers markets often indicate a 300% increase in SNAP and WIC use at farmers markets with the introduction of double voucher incentive programs.[234]

Recommendations

Recommendation 4.7: Provide economic incentives to increase production of healthy foods such as fruits, vegetables, and whole grains, as well as create greater access to local and healthy food for consumers. The upcoming reauthorization of programs governed by the Food, Conservation and Energy Act of 2008 provides another opportunity to strengthen Federal farm and food policy to help meet the needs of all Americans.

Recommendation 4.8: Demonstrate and evaluate the effect of targeted subsidies on purchases of healthy food through nutrition assistance programs. Through the Healthy Incentives Pilot, the Food, Conservation, and Energy Act of 2008 provided $20 million to determine if incentives provided to SNAP recipients at the point-of-sale increase the purchase of fruits, vegetables, or other healthful foods. The evaluation of this pilot, still in the early development stages, will offer solid evidence on whether a financial incentive can influence fruit and vegetable purchases and consumption.

Recommendation 4.9: Analyze the effect of state and local sales taxes on less healthy, energy-dense foods based on nutrient content or categories with low nutritional value (such as soft drinks, candy, snack foods, and fast foods).

Benchmarks of Success

By 2020, increase the availability of fruits and vegetables in the American food supply by 70%, or 450 pounds per person per year. In 2008, the American food supply included 643. 6 pounds of fruit and vegetables per person—about 251 pounds of fruit and 393 pounds of vegetables.[235] A recent USDA analysis suggested that to bring American diets into alignment with recommendations in the 2005 Dietary Guidelines, consumption of fruit would have to increase by 132%, and consumption of vegetables would have to increase by 31%.[236] The increased supply of fruit and vegetables needed to support these consumption changes would total 1,096 pounds per person—an increase of 453 pounds, or over 70%.

USDA prepares these estimates of fruit and vegetables in the food supply on an annual basis, drawing on data from a variety of government and private sources, including farm production and stocks information from the Census of Agriculture, trade information from the U.S. Census Bureau and USDA's Agricultural Marketing Service, and information on processed products from trade association reports. Per capita estimates are calculated using population estimates for that particular year.

C. Product Formulation

In addition to ensuring access to supermarkets and grocery stores, these stores must also provide healthy options at affordable prices. Consumer demand plays an essential role in the range of foods available, yet decisions that the food and agriculture industries make in responding to these demands determine what is on store shelves. Parts of the food industry are undertaking efforts to reformulate products, and through concerted efforts, the marketplace can move faster and farther. To address the obesity crisis, we must expand and accelerate efforts to reformulate products, particularly those aimed at kids, so they have less fat, salt, and sugar, and more of the nutrients children need.

It is easy for companies to take advantage of the human craving for sugary, fatty, salty foods by creating products that are sweeter, richer, and saltier than ever before. Doing so does not just respond to people's natural inclinations, it also helps shape them. This is particularly dangerous for our Nation's children, as these foods become embedded in their life-long eating habits.

There is another choice. Just as we can shape children's preferences for high-calorie, low-nutrient foods, we can also shape their preference for high-quality, healthier foods. Making this a reality requires a serious industry-wide commitment to provide parents with healthier food options at affordable prices.

The food industry has shown that it can respond to new consumer demands, including demands related to health and nutrition. In 2008, manufacturers introduced about 23,000 new products, with claims such as "natural," "fresh," "organic," "no preservatives," "low or no trans fat," and "high vitamin," used to market about 25% of these new products. [237] In the competition for health-conscious consumers, processed food manufacturers quadrupled the average number of new whole-grain products introduced between 2001 and 2006.[238]

Rather than finding creative ways to market existing products as healthy, we must develop new products proven to be healthy—products that help shape the health habits of an entire generation. Products like baby carrots and apple slices have proven appealing to children, as well as whole grains. Developing and marketing more of these products, as well as reducing sugar in items popular with children like flavored milk or yogurt, help children form healthy habits and ultimately, combat the obesity trend.

Recommendations

Recommendation 4.10: The food, beverage, and restaurant industries should be encouraged to use their creativity and resources to develop or reformulate more healthful foods for children and young people.

- Industries should be encouraged to shift product portfolios to promote new and reformulated child-oriented foods and beverages that are substantially lower in total calories, fats, salt, and added sugars, and higher in nutrient content. This should be informed by research about which products are favored by children, and in particular, by children at high risk for obesity.
- Restaurants should be encouraged to expand and actively promote healthier food, beverage, and meal options for children, and be attentive to the effects of plate and portion size, as noted in Chapter II.

Benchmarks of Success

Increase new product introductions that are consistent with dietary recommendations and substantially lower in total calories, fat, salt, and added sugars. Proprietary data sources can be used to monitor the number and percent of annual product introductions with healthier formulations, such as low fat, no trans fat, low or no sodium, low or no sugar, added calcium, or reduced calories per serving. Over time, it should be possible to monitor consumer purchases of these new product introductions to determine whether they have become a larger share of purchases and intake, using commercial data.

D. Hunger and Obesity

In 2008, approximately 49 million people, including 17 million children, live in households struggling to put enough food on the table. In over 500,000 households, children skipped meals or ate less than needed because of lack of resources.[239] Scholars are increasingly discussing the possible correlation between weight status and food insecurity. This association seems paradoxical, since food insecurity results from inadequate resources to purchase enough food and obesity is a consequence of consuming too much. Still, a number of studies have suggested a possible correlation between food insecurity and obesity, especially in women.[240]

This relationship may exist because the low cost of nutrient-poor, energy-dense foods promotes overconsumption of calories, leading to weight gain. To maintain adequate energy intake, people who must limit food costs may select lower-quality diets, consisting of high-energy, inexpensive foods. People eat fewer fruits and vegetables as food insecurity worsens. Food insecurity may also lead to various psychological and behavioral changes, such as a preoccupation with food, stress, depression, and physical limitations in adults—all of which can lead to an increased risk for obesity. In addition, because many food-insecure households receive assistance from one or more Federal nutrition assistance programs, it is important to consider whether these programs contribute to the obesity/food insecurity paradox, or help solve the paradox by providing access to healthier food, incentives for healthier choices, and effective nutrition education.

USDA administers 15 Federal nutrition assistance programs as our Nation's first line of defense against hunger, including those mentioned above—the Supplemental Nutrition Assistance Program (SNAP, formerly food stamps), the National School Lunch Program (NSLP), the School Breakfast Program (SBP), and the Special Supplemental Nutrition Program for Women, Infants, and Children (WIC). The Federal government will invest more than $80 billion in the national nutrition safety net in fiscal year 2010, subsidizing meals and food purchases for more than 1 in 4 Americans. One-half of all children will participate in SNAP alone at some point during their childhood, including 90% of Arican-American children. [241]

Given these programs' extensive reach, it is important that they be part of the solution to childhood obesity. Data from the National Health and Nutrition Examination Survey show that generally there are more similarities than differences in the nutrient intakes, diet quality, and food choices of program participants compared to the rest of the American population. [242] A thorough assessment of the research in this field shows that WIC and school lunch and breakfast programs do not contribute to childhood obesity.

It remains important to ensure that those who are eligible for and in need of assistance have ready access to these programs. While these programs serve millions of low-income Americans, some people who need benefits do not participate; over one-third of individuals eligible for SNAP do not participate,[243]and 40% of those eligible for WIC do not participate[244]. They may not be aware they are eligible, may not realize the size and value of benefits, or may find applying difficult or burdensome. Similarly, although meal programs exist in thousands of schools across the country, not all eligible children participate in the NSLP, and even fewer participate in the SBP. School lunch is served in around 100,000 schools, while the breakfast program is only available in 88,000 schools and almost two-thirds of children who eat a school lunch do not receive a school breakfast. Some bring healthy food from home, but others, especially in high schools, may forego a nutritious lunch or breakfast entirely.

Is Poor Diet a Low Income Problem?

In general, when one looks at both the food choices and the diet quality of nutrition program participants and other consumers, the similarities are more striking than the differences:

- A recent analysis of nutrition monitoring data (Cole et al , 2008), comparing the diets of participants in SNAP, WIC, and the school meals programs with nonparticipants and higher income consumers show that the diets of all groups fall far short of the *Dietary Guidelines for Americans.* All groups had very low intakes of whole grains, dark green and orange vegetables, and legumes, and high intakes of fat, saturated fat and added sugars.
- With regard to the shopping practices of SNAP participants specifically, consumer expenditure data suggest that they tend to buy the same categories of foods as other consumers These differences are minor even though families at the high end of the income distribution spend *over twice as much on food at home* as those at the low end.

Nonetheless, some differences do appear to be linked to income:

- In 2003-04, people in low-income families had significantly lower intakes of total vegetables, dark green and orange vegetables and legumes, and whole grains than did higher income families.
- People in low-income families, compared with their counterparts, had lower (i e more healthful) intakes of sodium than higher-income families.
- The only significant difference in the quality of *children's* diets by family income, as measured by the Healthy Eating Index, was that low-income children had a higher score for total vegetables. This may reflect low-income children's greater participation in the National School Lunch Program (Guenther et al. 2008).

In general, the critical lesson from this evidence is that while some income-linked factors, such as improved access to healthy options, hold promise to support and influence better diets, almost all Americans, no matter their income need to make significant changes in their eating behaviors to promote good health.

Sources: Cole, N , Fox, M K (2008) *Diet Quality of Americans by Food Stamp Participation Status: Data from the National Health and Nutrition* Examination Survey. Washington, DC: Abt Associates, Inc ; Guenther, P M , Juan, W , Mark, L , Hiza, H A , Fugwe, T , Lucas, R (2008) Diet Quality of Low-Income and Higher Income Americans in 2003-04 as Measured by the Healthy Eating Index-2005 *Nutrition Insight*, 42.

Recommendations

Recommendation 4.11: Increase participation rates in USDA nutrition assistance programs through creative outreach and improved customer service, state adoption of improved policy options and technology systems, and effective practices to ensure ready access to nutrition assistance program benefits, especially for children. Improved policies and effective practices include streamlined and more timely application process, greater use of broad-based categorical eligibility and direct certification, and reductions of barriers to participation such as finger imaging. Access to feeding programs for children throughout the year can also be expanded by engaging state, local, Tribal, community leaders, and partnerships with allied organizations, advocacy groups, and communities.

Benchmarks of Success

Increase participation among people eligible for SNAP benefits to 75% by 2015. USDA estimates annual participation rates based on the Annual Social and Economic Supplement to the Current Population Survey and administrative data on SNAP participants. The SNAP participation rate was 65. 8% in 2007.

Increase National School Lunch Program participation by 2 million additional children (up to 60% of all students) and School Breakfast Program participation by 3 million additional children (up to 25% of all students) by 2015. USDA monitors participation in the school meal programs through periodic reporting by State administering agencies; information on school enrollments is available annually from the U. S. Department of Education. In 2009, 56% of enrolled students participated in lunch and 20% participated in breakfast.

Key Questions for Future Research

Making research in this area a priority may help to identify the relationship between access and consumption of healthy foods, as well as the causal links between access and diet related health outcomes Key issues to address with future research investments include:

- The definition, measurement, and consequences of food deserts on food access, diet, and weight outcomes;
- The impact of improved access on dietary quality and obesity rates;
- How agricultural policy may affect food prices and obesity rates;
- The comparative efficacy of sales taxes and price subsidies on weight outcomes; and
- The effectiveness of price incentives, including supplements that increase the value of farmers' market purchases or incentives to promote the purchase of fruits, vegetables, and other healthful foods, especially for low-income populations;

In addition, there is need for tools proven to help communities assess their progress in helping residents eat healthy foods, increase their knowledge of potential steps to promote healthy eating and good nutrition among community residents, as well as identify and define influential actions. This includes tools that connect to and use existing databases (such those that track which products are being sold at grocery stores, through UPC codes) to help communities, industry, and policymakers assess progress in shifting toward increased consumption of healthy foods.

Finally, focusing investments in food technologies, research, and development may help to identify and produce new and reformulated child-oriented foods and beverages that are substantially lower in total calories, fats, salt, and added sugars.

V. INCREASING PHYSICAL ACTIVITY

Physical activity is an essential component of a healthy lifestyle. In combination with healthy eating, it can help prevent a range of chronic diseases, including heart disease, cancer, and stroke, the three leading causes of death.[245] Risk factors for these diseases can begin early in life and be mitigated early in life by adopting regular physical activity habits. Physical activity helps control weight, builds lean muscle, reduces fat, and contributes to a healthy functioning cardiovascular system, hormonal regulatory system, and immune system; promotes strong bone, muscle and joint development; and decreases the risk of obesity.[246] Research has also found that physical activity is related to improvements in mental health, helping to relieve symptoms of depression and anxiety and increase self-esteem.[247] In addition, some studies show that physical activity is correlated with improved academic achievement.[248]

According to the Physical Activity Guidelines for Americans, children and adolescents should participate in physical activity for at least 60 minutes every day. [249] The Physical Activity Guidelines, developed in 2008 by a committee of experts convened by the U.S. Department of Health and Human Services, provide science-based guidance for Americans ages six and older. They recommend that children's activity time include moderate to vigorous aerobic activity, muscle strengthening, and bone-strengthening exercises, and that young people should be encouraged to participate in age-appropriate, enjoyable, and diverse activities. There are many examples of physical activity, including not only team sports but also walking, biking, swimming, hiking, dancing, gardening, and many other group or individual activities. Recreational activities enjoyable to youth help ensure that they continue to engage in those activities. For example, a survey of Americans who participated in an outdoor activity found that 90% of them began doing so between the ages of five and 18.[250] Outdoor activities can be enjoyed in a variety of locations and are often less expensive, more accessible, and can foster life-long activity.

Children should have several opportunities to be active throughout the week and year round. Activity should be a normal part of a child's day, from walking or biking to and from school, where appropriate, to participating in a physical education class, to engaging in active games during recess, after school, or in the summer at home, in a park, or on a playground. All children benefit and gain enjoyment from physical activity, regardless of ability or disability status, gender, or athletic inclinations and talents. The benefits of physical activity extend beyond childhood too—young people who grow up physically active are more likely to be active adults. [251]

PHYSICAL ACTIVITY GUIDELINES FOR CHILDREN AND ADOLESCENTS

Children and adolescents should get 60 minutes (1 hour) or more of physical activity daily.

- **Moderate- or vigorous-intensity aerobic** physical activity (such as running, hopping, skipping, jumping rope, swimming, dancing, and bicycling) should comprise most of the 60 or more minutes a day Vigorous-intensity physical activity should be included at least 3 days a week.
- **Muscle-strengthening** physical activity (such as playing on playground equipment, climbing trees, playing tug-of-war, lifting weights, or working with resistance bands) should be included at least 3 days of the week.
- **Bone-strengthening** physical activity (such as running, jumping rope, basketball, tennis, and hopscotch) should be included at least 3 days of the week.

Young people should be encouraged to participate in physical activities that are appropriate for their age, that are enjoyable, and that offer variety For more information, see http://www health gov/paguidelines/

Young people who believe they are competent and have the skills to be physically active are more likely to be active. [252] Likewise, young people who feel supported by friends and families or are surrounded by others interested in physical activity, are more likely to participate in both structured and non-structured activities. [253] These social norms are powerful in determining people's actions.

Unfortunately, our young people live in a social and physical environment that makes it easy to be sedentary and inconvenient to be active. Social and environmental factors that discourage physical activity include: community design centered around automobiles, limited access to low or no cost physical activity close to home (such as parks, recreation centers, and walking and biking paths); new technology that is sedentary in nature; and increased concerns about safety in neighborhoods. The results are startling. Fewer than one in five high school students meet the current recommendations of 60 minutes of daily physical activity,[254] and a recent study showed that adolescents now spend more than seven hours per day watching television, DVDs, movies, or using a computer or a mobile device like a cell phone or MP3 player. [255] Older adolescents are less likely than younger children to be physically active, and adolescent girls are less likely to be physically active than their male peers. [256] African-American and Hispanic adolescent girls are the least likely to be physically active.

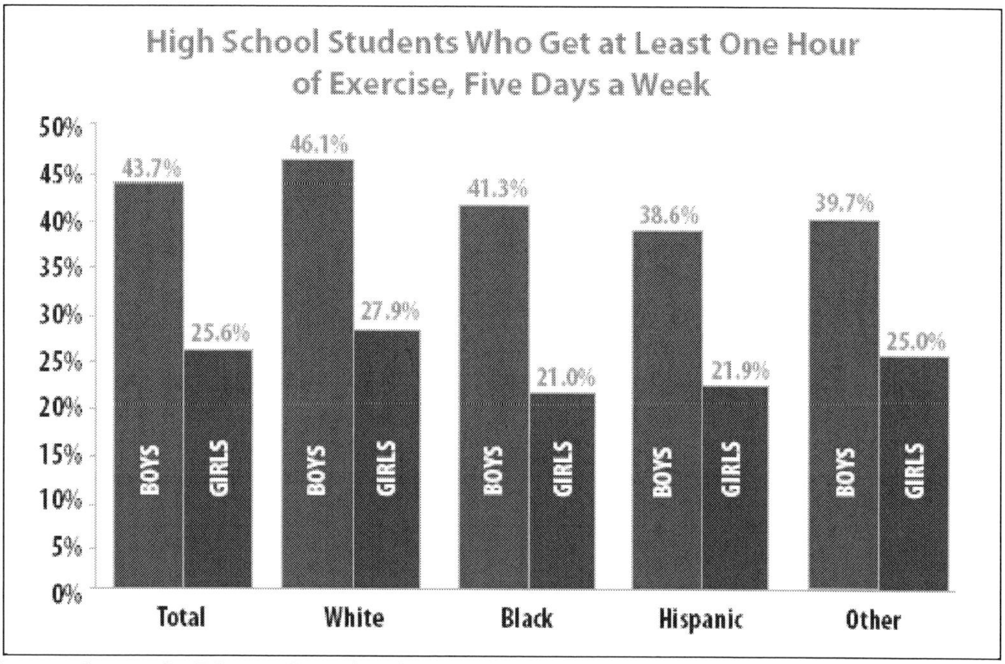

Source: Centers for Disease Control and Prevention's National Youth Risk Behavior Surveillance—United States, 2007.

COMMUNITY RESOURCES FOR ENGAGING YOUNG PEOPLE WITH DISABILITIES IN PHYSICAL ACTIVITY

BlazeSports America is a direct legacy of the 1996 Paralympic Games held in Atlanta, Georgia This organization, with school and community programs in all states, includes sports, camps, and athletic competitions that seek to increase independence, improve health, and enhance overall quality of life for youth and adults with physical disabilities The organization provides support and toolkits for schools and communities to help develop comprehensive programs and create opportunities for including students with disabilities in athletics and physical activity, including an equipment loan program With programs geared for individuals throughout the lifespan, BlazeSports provides programs and services that moves children and youth through a continuum, starting with lessons on active play and teaching lessons on being active for life More information on BlazeSports America can be found at:_httpi/www blazesports org

Another nonprofit organization, the National Center for Physical Activity and Disability, offers a searchable database of programs by geographic region for students with disabilities at: httpi/www ncpad org/programs/index-title php?letter=A

There are added barriers for vulnerable populations to become more physically active. Research shows that children with physical, sensory, and cognitive disabilities have substantially greater difficulty participating in regular physical activity, compared with the general population. A recent study showed that youth with physical disabilities had a 4.5 times higher rate of physical inactivity compared to youth without a disability, and they were twice as likely to report watching television for more than four hours per day.[257] Children with physical and developmental disabilities are significantly more likely to be obese or overweight compared with peers without disabilities of the same age.[258] However, there is growing awareness that many activity and health disparities reported among children and adults with disabilities are not necessarily a direct result of the disability, but rather a result of the challenges these individuals face in accessing community services and programs. Such challenges include poor accessibility of facilities, services, and programs, as well as environmental barriers such as lack of accessible equipment or transportation. To overcome these barriers and reduce disparities in physical activity, public schools must ensure that services, supports, and programs, including health and physical education programs, are equally accessible to eligible students with disabilities as to those without disabilities, pursuant to the Individuals with Disabilities Education Act (IDEA) and Title II of the Americans with Disabilities Act (ADA).[259] Many children who do not attend school or live in traditional community settings, such as those in juvenile detention and correctional centers, also have fewer opportunities for physical activity and consequently are less active.[260]

Much of the existing research suggests that coordinated, multi-component programs and policies are necessary to effectively change social norms, environments, and behaviors. [261] As part of a comprehensive approach to encourage young people to be more active, schools and communities should be encouraged to adopt common and consistent policies, practices, and expectations regarding these goals. They should also provide opportunities for healthy lifestyle choices in all childhood settings before, during, and after school, as well as on weekends, holidays, and school vacations. [262] This requires changes at all levels, including individual changes; choices, attitudes, and behaviors about physical activity; the structure of school days; teaching approaches; the physical environments of communities; and policy decisions that govern our way of life. [263] This chapter details what can be done to increase children's physical activity levels:

- in schools and in activities outside of school;
- in the community with the built environment;
- to improve the accessibility of parks and playgrounds; and
- in indoor and outdoor recreational settings.

A. School-Based Approaches

Schools are a key setting to focus on, given the significant portion of time children spend there. Schools can undertake a combination of strategies and approaches to help children be more active including:

- Creating infrastructure and policies that increase access to and encourage physical activity for all students;
- Collecting valid and reliable data and using analytical tools and systems to understand student needs and fitness levels, and promoting approaches that are effective in changing physical activity behaviors and, ultimately, health outcomes;
- Maintaining strong physical education (PE) programs that engage students in moderate to vigorous physical activity for at least 50% of PE class time;

- Providing a variety of activities and specific skills so that students can be physically active not just during class but throughout the day and year; and
- Providing qualified school professionals who are trained in teaching methods to engage students in PE, including for students who face greater barriers to activity.

Most physical activity for students can be provided through a comprehensive school-based physical activity program. Such a program is anchored in quality PE and complemented by activities before, during, and after school, as well as in recess, other physical activity breaks, intramural and physical activity clubs, interscholastic sports, and walk and bike to school initiatives. 264 These initiatives should not take the place of PE, but should reinforce lessons taught in PE by providing opportunities to practice and apply the skills learned. [265]

The components of a comprehensive physical activity program, as identified by the CDC and the National Association for Sport and Physical Education, are described in more detail below. Although the approach focuses on schools and school-related interventions, many community sectors play a role in design, implementation, or evaluation of these interventions.

Schools are an important setting because of access to young people and the school's influence on behavior, as well as the potential impact physical activity has on learning, cognition, and academic achievement. A recent study conducted by the CDC[266] reviewed all relevant literature on the impact on education-related outcomes of school-based PE, recess, classroom-based physical activity, and extracurricular physical activities. Their analysis found that spending time on these four physical activity approaches had either a positive effect on academic achievement or, at minimum, did not detract from academic outcomes. Specifically:

- Eleven of the 14 studies on school-based PE showed one or more positive associations between this intervention and indicators of academic performance;
- All eight studies on recess found one or more positive association between recess and indicators of cognition, emotion, and academic behaviors, as well as a positive or no effect on children's attention, concentration, and/or on-task classroom behavior;
- Eight of nine studies on classroom physical activity, either through physical activity breaks or learning activities designed to promote learning through physical activity, found positive associations between these activities and indicators of cognitive and academic behavior; and
- All 19 studies examining the relationship between participation in extracurricular physical activity, including afterschool sports or other afterschool physical activity programs, and academic performance found one or more positive associations.

Some school leaders have expressed concerns that a comprehensive physical activity program is too expensive, particularly during difficult economic times and tight budgets However, there are many low-cost or no-cost steps that school leaders can take to improve the physical activity environment for all students and to promote student health without compromising academic pursuits

Policies that Support a Comprehensive Physical Activity Program

Local wellness policies, required by USDA for all school districts participating in a school-based meal program, can be used to create district guidelines that can significantly impact physical activity requirements for students. There are many examples that individual school districts can draw from as they develop or refine their wellness policies. They range from specifying minutes of PE or recess requirements, to restrictions on the use of physical activity as punishment. For example, Michigan provides a model local wellness policy for its school districts, combining a quality PE program with a coordinated school health framework and presenting ideas such as recess before lunch and extra physical activity breaks as a reward instead of food snacks. [267] However, a recent nationwide study that assessed the effectiveness and relative quality of local wellness policies showed that only 18% of policies reviewed addressed recess and most did not address PE. Physical activity was often the weakest component of the wellness policies. [268]

Effective implementation of wellness policies is also critical. For example, a study conducted during the first year of local wellness policy implementation in rural Colorado revealed that policies were poorly or weakly worded, and ultimately, had little to no effect on physical activity. Competing pressures, lack of support and resources, and no monitoring or accountability were cited as reasons for the policies' relative weakness.[269]

Physical Education (PE)

Physical Education (PE) is considered the cornerstone of a school-based comprehensive physical activity program. It provides the basis and opportunity for young people to gain the knowledge and skills needed to maintain physically active lifestyles throughout childhood and into adulthood. A quality PE program can increase student participation in physical activity, increase their physical fitness,[270] and enhance their understanding about the purpose and methods of physical activity. [271] Participation in daily PE is associated with an increased likelihood of participating regularly in moderate to vigorous physical activity. [272]

The evidence strongly supports the correlation between school-based PE and increasing physical activity rates. The Task Force on Community Preventive Services is an independent, non-federal, volunteer body of public health and prevention experts tasked with reviewing evidence for interventions, providing recommendations that promote health, and identifying areas for further research. This group reviewed the literature and found that enhanced, school-based PE is an effective strategy for increasing physical activity among young people. [273]

The National Association for Sport and Physical Education recommends daily PE from kindergarten through grade 12, suggesting 150 minutes per week for elementary schools and 225 minutes per week for secondary schools. [274] Pursuant to their findings, a quality PE program should:

- meet the needs of all students;
- be an enjoyable experience for all students;
- keep students active for most of PE class time;
- teach self-management as well as movement skills; and
- emphasize knowledge and skills for a lifetime of physical activity. [275]

One of the resources available to school districts is the Physical Education Curriculum Analysis Tool (PECAT) issued by the CDC, which helps school districts conduct an analysis of their PE curriculum, based on national standards but with an option to customize to include local standards.

Effective school-based PE programs must also take into consideration children who are obese or who have physical or cognitive disabilities, chronic diseases (such as diabetes or asthma), or low levels of fitness. These children may need instruction in PE and physical activity programs to develop motor skills, improve physical fitness, and experience enjoyment and success. Nationwide, 62% of schools had students with long-term physical or cognitive disabilities or chronic diseases. Often, young people who have disabilities or chronic health conditions are discouraged from participating in PE class and other forms of physical activity. For example, among schools with students with physical disabilities, 59% allowed these students to be exempt from enrolling in PE.[276]

Influencing students' attitudes towards and perceptions of physical activity may affect their involvement in physical activity outside of PE class.[277] Physical education should encourage students to view physical activity as important and enjoyable. Increasing students' confidence in their ability to engage in physical activity increases the likelihood of enjoyment and therefore, the likelihood of regular participation in physical activity. [278] Students are more likely to have positive attitudes towards physical activity if their needs and interests are met through a variety of activities. They should also understand the many benefits of physical activity, and should be able to apply their newly acquired skills through various opportunities.

Outdoor Education through the Department of the Interior

Another strategy for getting kids physically active is to involve them in environmental education programs that involve outdoor activity. Interpretive programs and alternative PE lessons involving activities such as hiking, biking, wildlife watching, and kayaking can make outdoor education good for the body and brain, and at the same time, enhance young Americans' exposure to and appreciation of our nation's cultural, historic, and environmental resources. Additionally, the Fish and Wildlife Service and the National Park Service offer curriculum-based teacher training by field stations to classroom teachers and other educators to prepare their students for field trips to national parks, wildlife refuges, fish hatcheries, and other public lands. However, more can be done on the national level to encourage outdoor education on public lands as part of school-based curriculum. These programs also facilitate healthier lifestyles by emphasizing indoor and outdoor activity and exercise.

Another option for engaging students is to incorporate interesting PE lessons that make use of the natural environment. Outdoor education has an added advantage because students who become accustomed to outdoor activity are more likely to be active. [279] Depending on the climate, lessons can include activities as varied as hiking, canoeing, and snowshoeing.

Despite the evidence supporting PE, due to budget pressures and other factors, fewer than one in six schools require at least three days a week of PE for the entire school year for all grades in the school. Only 4% of elementary schools, 8% of middle schools, and 2% of high schools provide daily PE or its equivalent for the entire school year for all students.[280] While most middle schools and high schools require PE, 12% of middle schools and 25% of high schools allow students to be exempt from PE requirements because of participation in school sports. 14% of these middle schools and 20% of these high schools allow students to be exempt from PE for participation in school activities other than sports such as band or chorus.

For many schools, the barriers to incorporating PE during the school day include lack of time and resources, such as trained staff, and competing priorities. As noted above, research has shown that allowing students to participate in PE does not detract from academics[281] but rather may enhance academic achievement.[282]

Some states and school districts already require daily PE for students. Like local wellness policies though, unless these requirements are followed, they may not yield the intended results. In Florida, for example, the legislature enacted a requirement for 30 minutes of PE for elementary schools and daily PE for middle school students beginning in the 2009-10 school year. Some reports on thè effects of this policy show that school districts struggle to fully fund daily PE and classes are often too crowded to accommodate all students and meet the requirement.[283]

THE PROMISE OF TECHNOLOGY

Innovative and engaging teaching methods can motivate students to participate in PE, particularly those students who are not natural athletes or who do not enjoy "traditional PE." Some students have been motivated by the use of technology in the PE classroom that enhances individual skills and teaches students how to monitor their own fitness levels. Examples of technologies that have been incorporated into PE classrooms in recent years include heart rate monitors and equipment that combines activity with video or television-enabled games.

The promise of technology is still uncertain, however. Small, initial studies of these types of "exergaming" technologies suggest that these activities can help engage students who would not otherwise engage in activity and may burn more calories than being sedentary, but there are no studies yet showing a long-term effect on changing physical activity behaviors or on the overall impact on weight loss or children's health. Additionally, these technologies can be prohibitively expensive for school districts to buy and maintain.

Challenges and assessments can also be used to educate children and get them excited about being active. The President's Challenge (originally established in 1966 as the Presidential Physical Fitness Award) was created at the recommendation of the President's Council on Physical Fitness and Sports as a free, publicly-available tool intended both for assessment and engagement of children in fitness-enhancing activity. The Challenge has long provided fitness benchmarks for young people by means of a fitness test. However, the data that are used to classify young people into the three award categories are based on a nationwide sampling that may no longer be relevant, given the increased prevalence of overweight and obesity. While the original Challenge program focused primarily on measures of athletic performance, it has been expanded to include physical activity, in the form of the President's Council also administers the Presidential Active Lifestyle Award (PALA). PALA helps children and adults build healthy habits by committing to regular physical activity five days a week for six weeks. The First Lady's *Let's Move*! campaign has set a goal of doubling the number of children in the 2010-11 school year who earn a PALA award.

Recess for Elementary School Students, Physical Activity Breaks for Older Students

Regularly scheduled recess periods provide another opportunity for children to get part of their recommended 60 minutes of daily physical activity.284 Recess allows children to apply skills learned in PE (such as decision making, cooperation, conflict resolution, and continued motor skill development). [285] It should not, however, replace PE or be used to meet time requirements set in PE policies. Recess also can provide the opportunity for children to enhance cooperation and negotiation skills, as well as improve attentiveness, concentration, and time-on-task in the classroom. [286] In addition, if recess is scheduled before lunch, students are likely to eat more food, including healthier foods, helping schools meet other desirable goals as well. [287]

Nearly all elementary schools provide regularly scheduled recess for students in at least one grade, but 26% of all elementary schools do not provide regularly scheduled recess for students in all grades. [288] The average length of recess was slightly less than 30 minutes, with more minutes offered for younger students. However, schools with more students from low-income families are even less likely to offer recess to students.[289]

Incorporating Movement into Curriculum and Classroom Activities

Schools can offer students breaks for movement during the school day, such as an extra few minutes for students to stretch before the beginning of a class, or integrating activity and movement into lessons. Some schools might offer physical activity in the classroom as part of planned lessons that teach mathematics, language arts, and other academic subjects through movement. These types of activities contribute to students' accumulated physical activity during the school day. [290] In addition to promoting good health, physical activity within the regular classroom can enhance on-task classroom behavior of students[291] and establish a school environment that promotes regular physical activity.

Recommendations

Recommendation 5.1: Developers of local school wellness policies should be encouraged to include strong physical activity components, on par with nutrition components.

Recommendation 5.2: The President's Challenge should be updated to ensure consistency with the Physical Activity Guidelines for Americans and to ensure ease of use and implementation byschools. Private sector partners with an interest in physical activity should help enroll children in the Presidential Active Lifestyle Award program.

Recommendation 5.3: State and local educational agencies should be encouraged to increase the quality and frequency of sequential, age- and developmentally- appropriate physical education for all students, taught by certified PE teachers. Promising strategies include:

- Research-based curriculum and instructional methods that engage students in moderate to vigorous physical activity for at least 50% of PE class time;
- Instruction in a variety of lifetime fitness activities such as walking, hiking, snowshoeing, rock climbing, water sports, and biking as alternatives to team sports, which can also engage students in long-term outdoor recreation activities while helping to teach principles of activity.
- Partnership with private companies that support local educational agencies through the purchase of necessary equipment for PE classes.

Recommendation 5.4: State and local educational agencies should be encouraged to promote recess for elementary students and physical activity breaks for older students, and provide support to schools to implement recess in a healthy way that promotes physical activity and social skill development. Developers of teacher preparation programs should be encouraged to provide instruction on recess management and activity breaks for students. These can include in-service training to teachers and school professionals on actively engaging students, managing recess, and providing supervision during physical activity breaks, if appropriate.

Recommendation 5.5: State and local educational agencies should be encouraged to provide opportunities in and outside of school for students at increased risk for physical inactivity, including children with disabilities, children with asthma and other chronic diseases, and girls. For example, local educational agencies, schools, and teachers should include considerations for ensuring physical activity for students with disabilities in their Individualized Education Plans, pursuant to the IDEA and/or the ADA; State and local educational agencies should be encouraged to follow the National Guidelines for Managing Asthma at Schools;[292] and Title IX should be maintained and enforced to ensure gender equity.

Benchmarks of Success

Increase the number of high school students who participate in daily PE classes to 40% by 2015 and 50% by 2030. Currently, roughly 30% of high school students attend daily PE classes, a rate that has been relatively stable since about 1993. This data can be tracked using the national Youth Risk Behavior Survey. Note that while the quality of PE classes cannot be tracked with current survey instruments, the goal is to increase both quantity and quality. Similar progress for elementary students should be made, and can be tracked if data becomes available.

Increase the percentage of schools that offer recess to all students and grades in elementary schools to 95% in 2015. As of 2006, only 79% of schools offered recess to all of these students. Data are collected every six years through the CDC's School Health Policies and Practices Survey (SHPPS). The most recent SHPPS data is for 2006; the next study will be done in 2012 and released in 2013.

As noted earlier in this report, it will be critically important to monitor the overall increase in children's level of aerobic physical activity and muscle-strengthening activity. An enhanced NHANES survey may provide additional data on younger children's physical activity levels across the U.S. Additionally, the revamped President's Challenge tool may offer children, families, and teachers an understanding of how their physical activity performance has improved over time.

THE EXPANDED LEARNING TIME MODEL IN MASSACHUSETTS

Twenty-two schools in Massachusetts have received grants to adopt an expanding learning time model (ELT) and have incorporated more time for such activities through a variety of strategies including adding and/or expanding physical education classes; adding and/or expanding recess; and adding new health and fitness electives. These schools have also initiated a range of community partnerships with entities such as YMCAs, Boys & Girls Clubs, and community centers to connect youth in these schools to the organizations' staff and facilities.

For example, three middle schools in Boston that offer ELT offer a menu of health and fitness electives led by teachers and community partners, including a running club, step team, and competitive basketball, football, volleyball, and dance teams. The schools have established partnerships with the Boston Ballet to offer dance, partner with the Charlestown Community Center and Boston Centers for Youth and Families to offer swimming, and offer break-dancing in partnership with the Bird Street Community Center.

B. Expanded Day and Afterschool Activities

Expanded day and afterschool programs also offer schools an opportunity to collaborate with community partners to provide programming to many students. These programs can provide additional opportunities for learning, safe environments for students, and enrichment activities that integrate lessons about healthy living and additional opportunities for students to be active. Expanded day and afterschool activities can appeal to a variety of students' interests, ranging from instruction in such subjects as art and nutrition to engagement in intramural sports and non-competitive lifetime physical activities.

In the school setting, schools may rethink the length and structure of the school day and year, so students have the time they need to succeed, including through activities to improve their physical health, and teachers have the time they need to collaborate and improve their practice. While many of these schools have implemented an expanded day only recently, initial evidence suggests a positive relationship between expanded time programs and academic performance. [293] Research supports the effectiveness of well designed programs that expand learning time by a minimum of 300 hours per school year.[294] Research also demonstrates that students that participate in evidence-based afterschool programs improved participants social and personal skills, as well as academic achievement.[295]

Other activities during the after-school hours can enhance physical activity, including intramural sports and lifetime activities. The National Association for Sport and Physical Education has outlined three characteristics that describe the positive attributes of intramural sports programs: (1) students have a choice of activities or participation; (2) every student is given equal opportunity to participate regardless of ability level; and (3) students have the opportunity to be involved with the planning and implementation of activities.[296] Intramurals can offer students an opportunity to experiment and participate in new activities without having to try out for a team or playing in a high-pressure environment. Almost half of all schools in 2006 offered intramural programs. [297] Some intramural sports programs integrate academic content with physical activity or focus primarily on positive youth development, building social competencies, and connectedness between young people and adults. These types of programs, sometimes referred to as "sports-based youth development programs," focus on building students' social and emotional skills, enhancing positive relationships to peers and caring adults, developing youth leadership, and connecting with the broader community, with sports as the basis.

Lifetime physical activities such as walking, running, hiking, swimming, tennis, dancing, and biking can also be fun activities offered by programs and schools, including after-school programs. 298 Activities should provide opportunities for girls and boys; meet the needs of students at all levels of skills and physical abilities, particularly those that are not athletically gifted; and reflect student interest. Programs may combine these activities with other initiatives, such as community service or service learning programs that engage students in meaningful community work. And if schools do not go year around, many of the same program models could be used to increase physical activity in the summer.

The U.S. Department of Education's 21st Century Community Learning Centers Program provides support for afterschool activities to students. The latest U.S. Department of Education data show that the centers served about 1.5 million students in 2008 in almost 10,000 sites and received over $1 billion in FY 2010. While the vast majority of the programs (9 out of 10) operated in schools, school districts were only directly responsible for administering approximately 60% of the programs. The remaining 40% were administered by community-based organizations and other eligible entities, including institutions of higher education, nationally-affiliated non-profit organizations, and for-profit organizations.

SOCCER ASA BUILDING BLOCKFOR LEARNING

America SCORES is an after-school program that combines soccer, creative writing, and service learning. With affiliates across the country, a pilot study of the America SCORES Bay Area in San Francisco showed that participants in the program had statistically significant lowering of BMI. An unpublished national evaluation showed also showed that participants had an increased level of physical activity, increased reporting of feelings of self-confidence, self-efficacy, and enjoyment in learning, increased reporting of reading enjoyment and longer time reading independently, and gains in writing achievement.

Sources: Madsen K, Thompson H, Wlasiuk L, Queliza E, Schmidt C, Newman T (2009) After-school program to reduce obesity in minority children: A pilot Study *Journal of Child Health* Care, 13, 333; America SCORES Works (n d) Retrieved from: http://www americascores org/#/national/program/184

The Administration's Blueprint to reauthorize the Elementary and Secondary Education Act proposes to reform and strengthen 21st Century Community Learning Centers Program by incorporating approaches that better integrate community involvement and comprehensively redesign and expand the school day. In addition to providing additional time for academic work, programs would also explicitly focus on providing enrichment activities, including those that improve mental and physical health, opportunities for experiential learning, and greater chances for families to actively engage in their children's education.

Physical activity programs at the local level are often offered by a variety of providers, including park and recreation departments within local government, faith-based entities, or community centers like the YMCA or Boys and Girls Clubs. These outside partners can be of particular help in bringing in expertise and experience that might not always exist in schools or districts. Partnerships with parents and community-based organizations may increase the availability and quality of these programs, as well as the time students spend in physical activity. [299] They can also provide additional resources and supports.

In under-resourced communities, schools can provide the physical structure for after school, weekend, and summer programming. Community partners, with the support of local businesses or industry, can provide the personnel, programming, and support for activities. Some programs prefer to maintain relationships without formal agreements, while many others use more formalized agreements to delineate terms of the arrangement. Known as joint use agreements,[300] these arrangements can maximize the school facility and allow students to access playgrounds, gymnasiums, basketball courts, pools, or fields before and after school hours. In practice, these joint use agreements are also forged between schools and non-governmental entities, and include conditions and considerations for liability, a concern often cited by schools. A recent study showed that when a school ground was opened to children, not only were more children active as compared to a similar community, they also reported declines in watching television, DVDs, and movies, as well as playing video games on weekdays. [301]

All students, regardless of gender, race or ethnicity, health status, physical, sensory, or cognitive disability, should have access to physical activity programs. Physical activity programs that overemphasize team sports and do not emphasize lifetime physical activities can exclude potential participants.[302] As noted above in the discussion of PE, effective programs must also take into consideration children who are obese or who have physical or cognitive disabilities, chronic diseases (such as diabetes or asthma), or low levels of fitness. These children may need instruction to develop motor skills, improve physical fitness, and experience enjoyment and success.

Interscholastic Sports

Not surprisingly, participation in sports has been associated with higher levels of participation in overall physical activity.[303] One study suggested that adolescent participation in sports decreases cardiovascular risk factors, particularly for older adolescents. [304] Additionally, participation in sports programs has been associated with improved mental health and a reduction in risky health behaviors. [305] Girls in particular seem to benefit most from team sport participation; two recent studies suggested that girls who participated in athletics were healthier and had improved academic and career outcomes as adults. 306 Nationwide, 77% of middle schools and 91% of high schools offered interscholastic sports programs in 2006;[307] in 2007, 56% of high school students reported that they had played on at least one sports teams run by their school or a community group. [308] With the economic challenges facing school districts over the last few years, some administrators have cut or considered cutting team sports. Some research suggests that as much as $2 billion was cut from youth sport program budgets nationwide in 2008.[309] Other school districts have instituted "pay-to-play," which requires students to pay a fee to play on a sport team. According to a recent assessment by the National Federation of State High School Associations, 33 states have schools with pay-to-play programs. [310] A recent study showed that fees up to $100 cause a 10% decrease in participation, while fees up to $200 cause a 20% decline. [311] Costs can vary dramatically depending on the school district; in some districts, the price is capped and in others, participation is expensive. For example, in one district, it can cost as much as $282 to run cross-country, $508 to play field hockey, and $969 to play football. [312] For some students, particularly low-income students, this fee is impossible to pay and excludes students from engaging in sports.

Recommendations

Recommendation 5.6: Federal, state, and local educational agencies, in partnership with communities and businesses, should work to support programs to extend the school day, including afterschool programs, which offer and enhance physical activity opportunities in their programs.

- Districts, schools, local government, community-based organizations, and local businesses should partner together to create or enhance expanded day and afterschool programs that incorporate physical activity.
- Support should be provided to expand participation in intramural sports programs and non-competitive physical activity clubs that appeal to students who are not athletically gifted.
- Entities that accredit afterschool programs should include guidelines for incorporating age- and developmentally-appropriate physical activity in accreditation standards.
- State and local educational agencies should explore and execute joint use agreements to secure school facilities for out-of-school time activities and provide age- and developmentally- appropriate programming for students.
- The Federal government should support state, local educational agencies, and nonprofit organizations by providing resources, including funding and technical assistance, to promote high quality after school programs and programs that comprehensively redesign and expand the school schedule for all students, and full-service community schools through the 21st Century Community Learning Centers program. Technical assistance should also focus on innovative methods that ensure inclusive opportunities to promote physical activity for students with disabilities, as well as strengthening partnerships.

Recommendation 5.7: State and local educational agencies should be encouraged to support interscholastic sports and help decrease prohibitive costs of sports by curbing practices such as "pay-to-play," working with other public and private sector partners.

- The Federal government should continue to support programs, such as those sponsored by the Corporation for National and Community Service, that train and develop more qualified coaches for intramural sports teams and programs, and should collaborate with state, and local governments, nonprofits, philanthropies, and private sector partners to ensure that these programs are more widespread.

- State and local governments should consider strategies to make facilities and coaches more available for local youth sports teams.
- College and university sports teams should engage K-12 teams to increase opportunities for young people to learn about sports and receive coaching, and local sports figures and businesses should become more involved in supporting or sponsoring K-12 sports teams.

C. The"Built Environment"

How communities are designed and function can promote—or inhibit—physical activity for children and adults. The built environment consists of all man-made structures, including transportation infrastructure, schools, office buildings, housing, and parks. Children's ability to be physically active in their community depends on whether the community is safe and walkable, with good sidewalks and reasonable distances between destinations.

Research is still emerging on the exact interaction of the built environment and the impact on childhood obesity. Yet, a series of research studies suggests that attributes of our current built environment, such as low density development and sprawl, have had a negative impact on health outcomes, contributing to obesity and related health problems. [313] Several of these studies have found that areas with greater sprawl tend to have higher rates of adult obesity. The combination of greater distances between destinations as development sprawls outward from city centers and the lack of pedestrian and bicycle infrastructure contributes to eliminating walking and biking as options and to increased driving. One-fifth of all automobile trips in urban areas are one mile or less, and over two-fifths of these trips are under three miles,[314] distances easily walked or biked if the proper infrastructure were available. Low-income communities in particular often have a higher number of busy through streets, poor cycling and pedestrian infrastructure, and few high-quality parks and playgrounds—all elements which seem to deter physical activity.[315]

On the other hand, communities that emphasize pedestrian-friendly design have the potential to bring about better health outcomes. Such designs help decrease automobile travel, increase opportunities for physical activity, enhance public safety, and improve air quality, while simultaneously preserving agricultural and other environmentally fragile areas. Research suggests that doubling residential density across a metropolitan area might lower household vehicle miles traveled by about 5 to 12%, and perhaps by as much as 25%, if coupled with other measures. [316]

Creating new walkable, bikable communities can be feasible, but retrofitting the vast majority of existing American communities poses a separate challenge. This includes revitalizing older, traditional neighborhoods, often found in center cities or towns, to make them more viable, active communities. It also includes retrofitting newer sprawling communities to diversify their transportation options, creating a more walkable street grid.

Before undertaking any major new development or planning initiatives, communities may consider completing an assessment of the potential health impacts of the development. For example, Health Impact Assessments (HIAs) describe a combination of procedures, methods, and tools used to judge a policy or project's potential public health effects and the distribution of those effects within the population. [317] HIAs can be used to focus decision-makers' attention on the health consequences of the projects and policies they are considering, particularly how land use decisions may impede or improve physical activity.

The existence of safe, convenient, and accessible facilities for walking and biking are likely to increase physical activity and make parents feel more secure about their children's safety. However, they do not by themselves ensure more active lifestyles for residents of such communities. "Social environments" also play a role, including how community members feel about their neighborhood, how secure they feel, and how interested they are in participating in community-based physical activity. Evidence suggests that the combined effect of the built and social environment has an impact on rates of childhood obesity and overweight. A recent study found that:

- Children living in unsafe neighborhoods or those characterized by poor housing and the presence of garbage and litter on streets had an approximately 30-60% higher chance of being obese or overweight than children living in better conditions.
- Children with low neighborhood amenities or those lacking neighborhood access to sidewalks or walking paths, parks or playgrounds, or recreation or community centers had 20-45% higher odds of becoming obese or overweight compared to children who had access to these amenities.
- The impact of the built environment was particularly strong for younger children (ages 10-11) and for girls. Girls ages 10-11 living in neighborhoods with the fewest amenities had 121-276% higher adjusted odds of being obese or overweight than those living in neighborhoods with the most amenities. [318]

In particular, violence shapes our everyday decisions about where to live, work, go to school, shop for groceries, play, and whether go for a walk in the neighborhood or to a local park. In one study, people who classified their neighborhood as "not at all safe" were three times more likely to be physically inactive during leisure time than those who considered their neighborhood to be "extremely safe."[319] Another study also found that walking habits vary according to an individual's perception of safety and physical surroundings. For example, fear may lead someone to shop at a nearby convenience store, which may only contain unhealthy food, instead of walking further to a farmers market, or a grocery store that has healthy produce options. [320] Effective public safety measures, such as community based anti-crime and anti-gang initiatives, can reduce fear of crime and violence. Where possible, such efforts should be targeted on specific "hot spots" for crime and violence that impede access to parks, playgrounds, and other recreational facilities, as well as routes to healthy eating options.

"Active Transport": Safe Routes to School and Beyond

Active transport refers to approaches that encourage individuals to actively travel between their destinations throughout the day, such as by biking or walking. Children who walk or bike to school report being more physically active, including engaging in more moderate to vigorous physical activity, than those who travel by car, bus, or train. [321]

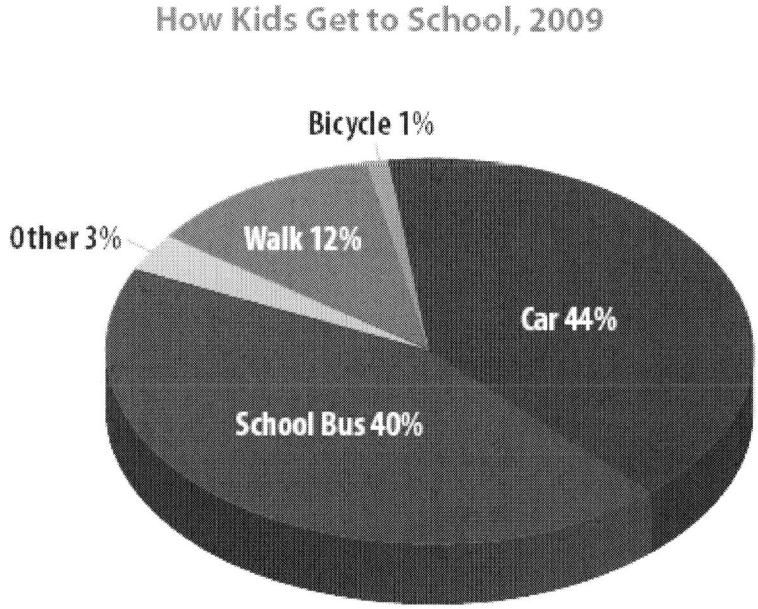

Source: U.S. Department of Transportation, Federal Highway Administration Office of Policy, National Household Travel Survey, 2009.

Programs like Safe Routes to Schools (SRTS), funded by the U.S. Department of Transportation (DOT), have proven an effective way to get students safely walking and biking to school. Serving students in grades K-8, the SRTS program supports capital investments, such as building sidewalks, crosswalks, creating better community designs, and providing other supports for active transport. Nearly 6,500 schools are participating in the federal SRTS program, which has provided $612 million for this purpose since 2005. SRTS helped and continues to help increase the number of students walking to school[322] and decrease those being driven to school. [323] A study of SRTS sites in California showed a 38% increase in students walking to school. [324]

Even without dedicated funding, some communities have found creative ways to make safe passages for young people between homes and neighborhoods, schools, and after school activities. For elementary students, the "walking school bus" has been a successful model, in which adults walk to school with a group of students. For older students, creative partnerships with police departments have helped students travel between school and afterschool activities safely in some communities.

Still, in 2009, only 13% of students rode a bike or walked to school, down from 44% in 1969. [325] Similarly, the percentage of students riding a school bus has also declined and more students report coming to school by personal vehicle than other methods. [326] Parents cite many barriers to "active transport," commonly referencing distance to school, traffic-related danger, and weather. In the same survey, 12% of parents cited fear of crime as a barrier. Six percent of parents also cited school policies that prohibit walking and biking to school as the reason their children did not walk or bike to school. 327 Bike and pedestrian safety is a real concern as well. In 2007, 14,000 children were injured and 300 killed by cars. There is a "safety in numbers" trend, in which roadways generally become safer for everyone when more people are out walking and biking.[328]

Recommendations

Recommendation 5.8: Reauthorize a Surface Transportation Act that enhances livability and physical activity. A complete network of safe bicycle and pedestrian facilities would allow children to take more trips through active transportation and get more physical activity. New Federal aid construction projects should accommodate bicyclists and pedestrians by incorporating "Complete Streets" principles. As improvement projects for existing facilities are undertaken, transportation infrastructure should be retrofitted, where feasible, to support and encourage bicycle and pedestrian use. State and local money can also be leveraged to support safe facilities for children to walk or bike to places like parks, playgrounds, transit, and community centers. The reauthorization could adopt Complete Streets principles that would include routine accommodation of walkers and bicyclists for new construction, to influence retrofitting of existing communities, and to support public transportation. In addition, it could enhance authority for recreational areas on public lands.

Recommendation 5.9: The Environmental Protection Agency should assist school districts that may be interested in siting guidelines for new schools that consider the promotion of physical activity, including whether students will be able to walk or bike to school.

Recommendation 5.10: Communities should be encouraged to consider the impacts of built environment policies and regulations on human health. Local communities should consider integrating Health Impact Assessments (HIAs) into local decision-making processes, and the Federal government should continue to support the development of an HIA approach, tools, and supporting resources that promote best practices.

Recommendation 5.11: The Federal Safe Routes to School Program (SRTS) should be continued and enhanced to accommodate the growing interest in implementing Safe Routes to Schools plans in communities. This can be facilitated by:

- Continuing aspects of current law, including requiring that every State maintain a full-time SRTS Coordinator, spending funds on both infrastructure projects and non-infrastructure activities, and continuing to operate the National Clearinghouse.
- Continuing Federal investments to increase opportunities for SRTS participation.
- Streamlining Federal requirements and reducing administrative burden for grants management to fit with the unique nature of SRTS projects and programs.
- Expanding funding eligibility to cover kindergarten through 12th grade.
- Developing improved surveillance and validated measures for tracking participation in SRTS and its impacts.

Recommendation 5.12: "Active transport" should be encouraged between homes, schools, and community destinations for afterschool activities, including to and from parks, libraries, transit, bus stops, and recreation centers.

Benchmarks of Success

Increase by 50% by 2015 the percentage of children ages 5-18 taking safe walking and biking trips to and from school. An increase of 50% would mean that 19 5% of school trips would be by biking or walking. This data is available from the National Household Travel Survey, which is conducted every five to seven years, so there may be a delay in this data becoming available.

D. Community Recreation Venues

Parks and Playgrounds

Parks and playgrounds in a community can provide opportunities to run and play and may increase unstructured physical activity.[329] If children can easily access safe parks and playgrounds in good repair, they are more likely to engage in recreational physical activity there.[330]

National, state, and local parks are an ideal environment to be physically active, and increased access to parks is proven to promote physical activity among children[331] and adolescents.[332] In addition to encouraging physical activity, parks and other natural landscapes can provide recreational experiences, opportunities to learn and grow, and places of quiet refuge. The Federal government provides support for state and local conservation and recreation initiatives through the Land and Water Conservation Fund (LWCF) State Assistance Program. The goal of this program is to increase access to a park, a river, or an area of open space close to home. As part of this initiative, funds can be used to enhance and support the further development of parks and playgrounds in communities. Other Federal programs provide funding to States and local entities for park and open space conservation and recreation trails and shared use paths, including HUD's Community Development Block Grant program and DOT's Transportation Enhancement program.

Private, nonprofit organizations and corporations have also supported park and playground development in communities. By engaging in park clean-ups and playground development, businesses can take part in initiatives that contribute to community cohesion and improve access to playgrounds and parks.

Outdoor and Indoor Venues

Outdoor recreation and access to nature play a vital role in the physical, psychological, spiritual well-being, health, and development of people of all ages.[333] The current poor health of many American children today, including increasing levels of obesity-related illnesses,[334] attention deficit- hyperactivity, vitamin D deficiency, and myopia are being attributed, in part, to a generational decline in the level of outdoor recreation in natural environments.

Children's level of physical activity has been shown to increase when they participate in environmental education programs that promote outdoor activity.[335] Children of all ages are healthier, happier, and have better social skills if they have frequent opportunities for free and unstructured play outdoors.[336] For these reasons, children need to be encouraged to connect with the outdoors—places that can promote both physical and emotional health.

Communities still need to ensure adequate and accessible indoor facilities for physical activity. For students who are unable to play outside because of allergies or asthma, particularly during high-pollution days or inclement weather, communities should make sure indoor recreational facilities are available to children. Currently, 65% of schools allow for community use of physical activity or athletic facilities, a strategy that can increase opportunities for indoor activity. [337]

Communities also must ensure that children actually are aware of the opportunities available to them. The Task Force for Community Preventive Services found that informational outreach is essential to maximizing the results of improvements in access to physical activity. [338] In some communities, outreach was unnecessary, but in others, outreach and communications was needed.

Recommendations

Recommendation 5.13: Increase the number of safe and accessible parks and playgrounds, particularly in underserved and low-income communities. This can be accomplished in part by:

- Targeting LWCF funds to increase use of and access to parks and open space in low-income neighborhoods and communities that receive funding, and by expanding Tribes' access to funding and strengthening their capacity to compete for funding.
- Businesses considering "adopting" (building and/or helping to maintain) parks and playgrounds in their communities.
- Foundations, community and faith-based organizations, and businesses engaging in community planning efforts to ensure their work in developing parks and playgrounds are enhanced and maintained over time, and are supportive of other community initiatives.
- Encourage development or renovation of playgrounds to include less asphalt and more natural terrain, so as to foster unstructured, "natural" play.

Recommendation 5.14: The Federal government should continue to support investments in a wide range of outdoor recreation venues, such as National Parks, Forests, Refuges and other public lands, and expand opportunities for children to enjoy these venues. The U. S. Department of Interior and the National Forest Service maintain hundreds of millions of acres of public land, as well as rivers, parks, and other areas.

- Federal land management agencies should work together along with state, Tribal and local agencies to promote and ensure access to a range of youth-appropriate activities on public lands and waters. This includes transportation to help children get to and from parks and other public lands.
- Federal agencies should work with non profits, corporations, and local youth groups to strengthen partnerships and identify new opportunities for outdoor physical activities, programs, and events.

Recommendation 5.15: Local governments should be encouraged to enter into joint use agreements to increase children's access to community sites for indoor and outdoor recreation.

Recommendation 5.16: The business sector should be encouraged to consider which resources and physical assets like fields and gyms can be used to increase students' access

to outdoor and indoor recreational venues. Corporations, for example, may have large grounds that they can make available for children in the community to play soccer or engage in other outdoor activities.

Recommendation 5.17: Entertainment and technology companies should continue to develop new approaches for using technology to engage children in physical activity.

Benchmarks of Success

Increase access to, use of, and the number of safe and accessible parks and playgrounds, particularly in underserved and low-income communities. Partial data sources exist in the private sector to measure this, but work will need to be done to develop those sources and measure progress.

Key Questions for Future Research

- What are the teaching methods that best engage students in PE, including the relative benefits of technology in the PE classroom, for achieving long-term behavioral changes in physical activity habits?
- What kinds of outdoor activities for children are most likely to produce lasting increases in physical activity levels? Are the benefits different from indoor physical activity?
- How can we better target physical activity interventions to multiple communities, including diverse ethnic populations and children with disabilities? What are the most effective methods for reaching these populations?
- What are appropriate measurement tools for tracking trends in physical activity?
- Do health impact assessments change health outcomes in communities where they are used?
- What percentage of children lives within walking or biking distance from school or a park entrance?
- Does the built environment increase physical activity rates for children and reduce obesity? If so, what are the mechanisms for this reduction?
- How can the insights of behavioral economics, such as changing the default choice in a given situation, be used to promote physical activity among young people?

CONCLUSION

Taken together, the strategies and tactics outlined in this report should achieve the goal of solving the problem of childhood obesity within a generation. It will not be easy, and it will take action on all of our parts — parents and teachers, leaders in government and industry, and communities large and small. But at the core of this endeavor is a simple concept we all embrace, which is that children should have good, nutritious food to eat and the chance to be physically active every day, so that they grow up into healthy adults.

The next step is to turn these ideas into action. Many partners stand ready to make this happen, and have already volunteered to be part of this effort by joining the First Lady's Let's Move! campaign. Philanthropies will play a critical role in cementing private sector commitments to make concrete steps towards our shared goal, including but not limited to the action steps recommended in this report. And the Federal government must play a leadership role as well. The Task Force on Childhood Obesity and its 12 member agencies stand ready to take up that charge. Every day, approximately 11,000 children are born in America. We owe them our very best effort.

SUMMARY OF RECOMMENDATIONS.

I. Early Childhood				
Recommendation	**Federal action**	**State or local action**	**Private sector action**	**Page**
Recommendation 1. 1: Pregnant women and women planning a pregnancy should be informed of the importance of conceiving at a healthy weight and having a healthy weight gain during pregnancy, based on the relevant recommendations of the Institute of Medicine.	x	x	x	12
Recommendation 1. 2: Education and outreach efforts about prenatal care should be enhanced through creative approaches that take into account the latest in technology and communications. Partners in this effort could include companies that develop technology-based communications tools, as well as companies that market products and services to pregnant women or prospective parents.			x	12
Recommendation 1. 3: Hospitals and health care providers should use maternity care practices that empower new mothers to breastfeed, such as the Baby-Friendly hospital standards.	x	x	x	16
Recommendation 1. 4: Health care providers and insurance companies should provide information to pregnant women and new mothers on breastfeeding, including the availability of educational classes, and connect pregnant women and new mothers to breastfeeding support programs to help them make an informed infant feeding decision	x	x	x	16
Recommendation 1. 5: Local health departments and community-based organizations, working with health care providers, insurance companies, and others should develop peer support programs that empower pregnant women and mothers to get the help and support they need from other mothers who have breastfed	x	x	x	16
Recommendation 1. 6: Early childhood settings should support breastfeeding	x	x	x	16
Recommendation 1.7: Federal and State agencies conducting health research should prioritize research into the effects of possibly obesogenic chemicals.	x			17
Recommendation 1.8: The AAP guidelines on screen time should be made more available to parents, and young children should be encouraged to spend less time using digital media and more time being physically active.		x	x	18

I. Early Childhood				
Recommendation 1.9: The AAP guidelines on screen time should be made more available in early childhood settings.		X	X	18
Recommendation 1.10: The Federal government, incorporating input from health care providers and other stakeholders, should provide clear, actionable guidance to states, providers, and families on how to increase physical activity, improve nutrition, and reduce screen time in early child care settings.	X			21
Recommendation 1.11: States should be encouraged to strengthen licensing standards and Quality Rating and Improvement Systems to support good program practices regarding nutrition, physical activity, and screen time in early education and child care settings		X	X	21
Recommendation 1.12: The Federal government should look for opportunities in all early childhood programs it funds (such as the Child and Adult Care Food Program at USDA, the Child Care and Development Block Grant, Head Start, military child care, and Federal employee child care) to base policies and practices on current scientific evidence related to child nutrition and physical activity, and seek to improve access to these programs	X			21
II. Empowering Parents and Caregivers Recommendation				
Recommendation 2.1: The Federal government, working with local communities, should disseminate information about the 2010 Dietary Guidelines for Americans through simple, easily actionable messages for consumers and a next generation Food Pyramid.	X			26
Recommendation 2.2: The FDA and USDA's Food Safety and Inspection Service should collaborate with the food and beverage industry to develop and implement a standard system of nutrition labeling for the front of packages.	X		X	27
Recommendation 2.3: Restaurants and vending machine operators subject to the new requirement in the Affordable Care Act should be encouraged to begin displaying calorie counts as soon as possible			X	27
Recommendation 2.4: Restaurants should consider their portion sizes, improve children's menus, and make healthy options the default choice whenever possible.			X	27
Recommendation 2.5: The food and beverage industry should extend its self-regulatory program to cover all forms of marketing to children, and food retailers should avoid in-store marketing that promotes unhealthy products to children.			X	32
Recommendation 2.6: All media and entertainment companies should limit the licensing of their popular characters to food and beverage products that are healthy and consistent with science-based nutrition standards.			X	32
Recommendation 2.7: The food and beverage industry and the media and entertainment industry should jointly adopt meaningful, uniform nutrition standards for marketing food and beverages to children, as well as a uniform standard for what constitutes marketing to children.			X	32
Recommendation 2.8: Industry should provide technology to help consumers distinguish between advertisements for healthy and unhealthy foods and to limit their children's exposure to unhealthy food advertisements.	X		X	32
Recommendation 2.9: If voluntary efforts to limit the marketing of less healthy foods and beverages to children do not yield substantial results,	X			32
II. Empowering Parents and Caregivers Recommendation				
the FCC could consider revisiting and modernizing rules on commercial time during children's programming.				

Summary of Recommendations (Continued).

Recommendation 2.10: Pediatricians should be encouraged to routinely calculate children's BMI and provide information to parents about how to help their children achieve a healthy weight.			x	35
Recommendation 2.11: Federally-funded and private insurance plans should cover services necessary to prevent, assess, and provide care to overweight and obese children.	x		x	35
Recommendation 2.12: Dentists and other oral health care providers should be encouraged to promote healthy habits and counsel families on childhood obesity prevention as part of routine preventive dental care			x	35
Recommendation 2.13: Medical and other health professional schools, health professional associations, and health care systems should ensure that health care providers have the necessary training and education to effectively prevent, diagnose, and treat obese and overweight children			x	35
III. Healthier Food in Schools Recommendation				
Recommendation 3.1: Update Federal nutritional standards for school meals and improve the nutritional quality of USDA commodities provided to schools.	x			39
Recommendation 3.2: Increase resources for school meals.	x	x	x	40
Recommendation 3.3: USDA should continue its outreach and technical assistance to help provide training for school food service professionals.	x	x	x	40
Recommendation 3.4: Schools should consider upgrading their cafeteria equipment to support the provision of healthier foods, for example, by swapping out deep fryers for salad bars.	x	x	x	41
Recommendation 3. 5: USDA should work with all stakeholders to develop innovative ways to encourage students to make healthier choices.	x	x		41
Recommendation 3.6: USDA should work to connect school meals programs to local growers, and use farm-to-school programs, where possible, to incorporate more fresh, appealing food in school meals.	x	x	x	41
Recommendation 3.7: Schools should be encouraged to make improvements in their school meal programs through the HealthierUS Schools Challenge in advance of updated Federal standards.	x	x	x	42
Recommendation 3.8: Increase the alignment of foods sold at school, including in the a la carte lines and vending machines, with the Dietary Guidelines.	x			43
Recommendation 3.9: Food companies should be encouraged to develop new products and reformulate existing products so they meet nutritional standards based on the Dietary Guidelines and appeal to children.			x	43
Recommendation 3.10: USDA and the U S Department of Education should collaborate with states to increase the availability and consis- tency of nutrition education in schools.	x	x		44
Recommendation 3.11: Where possible, use school gardens to edu- cate students about healthy eating.		x	x	45
Recommendation 3.12: Technical assistance should be provided to schools about how to a cafeteria and lunch room environment can support and encourage a healthful meal		x		45
Recommendation 3.13: Schools should be encouraged to ensure that choosing a healthy school meal does not have a social cost for a child		x		45
Recommendation 3.14: Schools should be encouraged to consider the impact of food marketing on education.		x	x	45

III. Healthier Food in Schools Recommendation				
Recommendation 3.15: School districts should be encouraged to cre- ate, post, and implement a strong local school wellness policy.	x	x	x	45
Recommendation 3.16: Promote good nutrition through afterschool programs.	x	x	x	47
Recommendation 3.17: Promote healthy behaviors in juvenile cor- rectional and related facilities.	x	x	x	47
IV. Access to Healthy, Affordable Food Recommendation				
Recommendation 4.1: Launch a multi-year, multi-agency Healthy Food Financing Initiative to leverage private funds to increase the availability of affordable, healthy foods in underserved urban and rural communities across the country.	x	x	x	53
Recommendation 4. 2: Local governments should be encouraged to create incentives to attract supermarkets and grocery stores to under- served neighborhoods and improve transportation routes to healthy food retailers.		x		54
Recommendation 4.3: Food distributors should be encouraged to explore ways to use their existing distribution chains and systems to bring fresh and healthy foods into underserved communities.	x		x	54
Recommendation 4.4: Encourage communities to promote efforts to provide fruits and vegetables in a variety of settings and encourage the establishment and use of direct–to-consumer marketing outlets such as farmers' markets and community supported agriculture subscriptions.		x		54
Recommendation 4.5: Encourage the establishment of regional, city, or county food policy councils to enhance comprehensive food system policy that improve health.		x		54
Recommendation 4.6: Encourage publicly and privately-managed facilities that serve children, such as hospitals, afterschool programs, recreation centers, and parks (including national parks) to imple- ment policies and practices, consistent with the Dietary Guidelines, to promote healthy foods and beverages and reduce or eliminate the availability of calorie-dense, nutrient-poor foods.	x	x	x	54
Recommendation 4.7: Provide economic incentives to increase production of healthy foods such as fruits, vegetables, and whole grains, as well as create greater access to local and healthy food for consumers.	x			59
Recommendation 4.8: Demonstrate and evaluate the effect of targeted subsidies on purchases of healthy food through nutrition assistance programs.	x			59
Recommendation 4.9: Analyze the effect of state and local sales taxes on less healthy, energy-dense foods.	x	x		59
Recommendation 4.10: The food, beverage, and restaurant industries should be encouraged to use their creativity and resources to develop or reformulate more healthful foods for children and young people.			x	60
Recommendation 4.11: Increase participation rates in USDA nutrition assistance programs through creative outreach and improved customer service, state adoption of improved policy options and technology systems, and effective practices to ensure ready access to nutrition assistance program benefits, especially for children.	x	x	x	62
V. Increasing Physical Activity Recommendation				
Recommendation 5.1: Developers of local school wellness policies should be encouraged to include strong physical activity components, on par with nutrition components.		x		73

Summary of Recommendations (Continued).

V. Increasing Physical Activity Recommendation				
Recommendation 5.2: The President's Challenge should be updated to ensure consistency with the Physical Activity Guidelines for Americans and to ensure ease of use and implementation by schools. Private sector partners with an interest in physical activity should help enroll children in the Presidential Active Lifestyle Award program.	X		X	73
Recommendation 5.3: State and local educational agencies should be encouraged to increase the quality and frequency of sequential, age- and developmentally- appropriate physical education for all students, taught by certified PE teachers.		X	X	73
Recommendation 5.4: State and local educational agencies should be encouraged to promote recess for elementary students and physical activity breaks for older students, and provide support to schools to implement recess in a healthy way that promotes physical activity and social skill development.		X		73
Recommendation 5.5: State and local educational agencies should be encouraged to provide opportunities in and outside of school for students at increased risk for physical inactivity, including children with disabilities, children with asthma and other chronic diseases, and girls		X	X	74
Recommendation 5.6: Federal, state, and local educational agencies, in partnership with communities and businesses, should work to support programs to extend the school day, including afterschool programs, which offer and enhance physical activity opportunities in their programs	X	X	X	77
Recommendation 5.7: State and local educational agencies should be encouraged to support interscholastic sports and help decrease prohibitive costs of sports by curbing practices such as "pay-to-play," working with other public and private sector partners.	X	X	X	78
Recommendation 5.8: Reauthorize a Surface Transportation Act that enhances livability and physical activity.	X	X		81
Recommendation 5.9: The Environmental Protection Agency should assist school districts that may be interested in siting guidelines for new schools that consider the promotion of physical activity, including whether students will be able to walk or bike to school	X	X		81
Recommendation 5.10: Communities should be encouraged to consider the impacts of built environment policies and regulations on human health	X	X		81
Recommendation 5.11: The Federal Safe Routes to School Program (SRTS) should be continued and enhanced to accommodate the growing interest in implementing Safe Routes to Schools plans in communities.	X			82
Recommendation 5.12: "Active transport" should be encouraged between homes, schools, and community destinations for afterschool activities, including to and from parks, libraries, transit, bus stops, and recreation centers.		X	X	82
Recommendation 5.13: Increase the number of safe and accessible parks and playgrounds, particularly in underserved and low-income communities	X	X	X	83
Recommendation 5.14: The Federal government should continue to support investments in a wide range of outdoor recreation venues, such as National Parks, Forests, Refuges and other public lands, and expand opportunities for children to enjoy these venues.	X			84
Recommendation 5.15: Local governments should be encouraged to enter into joint use agreements to increase children's access to com- munity sites for indoor and outdoor recreation.		X		84

V. Increasing Physical Activity Recommendation				
Recommendation 5.16: The business sector should be encouraged to consider which resources and physical assets like fields and gyms can be used to increase students' access to outdoor and indoor recreational venues.			x	84
Recommendation 5.17: Entertainment and technology companies should continue to develop new approaches for using technology to engage children in physical activity.			x	84

End Notes

[1] Ogden, C.L., Carroll, M., Curtin, L., Lamb, M., Flegal, K. (2010). Prevalence of High Body Mass Index in US Children and Adolescents 2007-2008. *Journal of American Medical Association, 303*(3), 242-249.

[2] Flegal, K.M., Graubard, B.I., Williamson D.F., et al. (2005). Excess deaths associated with underweight, overweight, and obesity. *Journal of the American Medical Association, 293*(15), 1861-7.

[3] Centers for Disease Control and Prevention, National Center for Health Statistics. (2007). National Diabetes Surveillance System. Incidence of Diabetes: Crude and Age-Adjusted Incidence of Diagnosed Diabetes per 1000 Population Aged 18-79 Years, United States, 1997–2004. Retrieved April 17, 2007 from: http://www.cdc.gov/diabetes

[4] Olshansky, J., Passaro, D., Hershow, R., Layden, J. et al. (2005, May 17). A Potential Decline in Life Expectancy in the United States in the 21st Century. *The New England Journal of Medicine, 352*(11), 1138- 1144.

[5] Finkelstein, E., Trogdon, J., Cohen J., Dietz, W. (2009). Annual Medical Spending Attributable to Obesity: Payer-And Service-Specific Estimates. *Health Affairs, 28*(5).

[6] Finkelstein, E., Trogdon, J., Cohen J., Dietz, W. (2009). Annual Medical Spending Attributable to Obesity: Payer-And Service-Specific Estimates. *Health Affairs, 28*(5).

[7] Trasande, L., Chatterjee, S. (2009). Corrigendum: The Impact of Obesity on Health Service Utilization and Costs in Childhood. *Obesity, 17*(9).

[8] Mission: Readiness – Military Leaders for Kids. (2010). *Too Fat to Fight: Retired Military Leaders Want Junk Food Out of America's Schools.* New York: Mission Readiness.

[9] Statement made by Curtis Gilroy, Director for Accession Policy. Office of the Under Secretary of Defense for Personnel & Readiness. Eismer, T. (2009, November 5). *New report reveals that 75% of young Americans are unfit for military service.* Mission: Readiness. [Press Release]. Retrieved from: http://cdn.missionreadiness.org/NATPR1109.pdf

[10] BMI is calculated by dividing a person's weight in kilograms by the height in meters squared.

[11] Prentice A.M., Jebb, S.A. (2001). Beyond body mass index. *Obesity, 2*(3), 141-7.

[12] National Institutes of Health. (1998). Clinical Guidelines on the Identification, Evaluation, and Treatment of Overweight and Obesity in Adults. The Evidence Report. *Obesity Research, 6*(supplement 2), 51S-209S

[13] U.S. Department of Health and Human Services. (2010). *The Surgeon General's Vision for a Healthy and Fit Nation.* Rockville, MD: U.S. Department of Health and Human Services, Office of the Surgeon General. Retrieved from http://www.surgeongeneral.gov/library/obesityvision/obesityvision2010.pdf.

[14] Ogden C.L., Flegal K.M., Carroll M.D, et al. (2002). Prevalence and trends in overweight among US children and adolescents, 1999-2000. *Journal of the American Medical Association, 288*(14), 1728-32; Ogden C.L., Carroll M.D., Curtin LR, et al. (2010). Prevalence of high body mass index in US children and adolescents, 200 7-2008. *Journal of the American Medical Association, 303*(3); 242-9.

[15] Ogden C.L., Carroll M.D., Curtin LR, et al. (2010). Prevalence of high body mass index in US children and adolescents, 2007-2008. *Journal of the American Medical Association, 303*(3), 242-9.

[16] Ogden C.L., Carroll M.D., Curtin LR, et al. (2010). Prevalence of high body mass index in US children and adolescents, 2007-2008. *Journal of the American Medical Association, 303*(3), 242-9.

[17] Anderson S.E., Whitaker R.C. (2009). Prevalence of obesity among US preschool children in different racial and ethnic groups. *Archives of Pediatrics and Adolescent Medicine, 163*(4), 344-8.

[18] Chang V.W., Lauderdale D.S. (2005). Income disparities in body mass index and obesity in the United States, 1971-2002. *Archives of Internal Medicine, 165*(18), 2122-8.

[19] Ogden C.L., Yanovski S.Z., Carroll M.D., et al. (2007). The epidemiology of obesity. *Gastroenterology, 132*(6), 2087-102.

[20] Pleis J.R., Lucas J.W., Ward B.W. (2009). Summary health statistics for U.S. dults: National Health Interview Survey, 2008. *Vital and Health Statistics. Series, 10*(242). Washington, D.C.: Government Printing Office.

[21] Ogden, C.L., Connor G.S., Rivera, Dommarco J, et al. (201 0). The Epidemiology of Childhood Obesity in Canada, Mexico and the United States. In L. Moreno, I. Pigeot and W. Ahrens (Eds.), *Epidemiology of*

obesity in children and adolescents - Prevalence and etiology. New York: Springer; Chang V.W., Lauderdale D.S. (2005). Income disparities in body mass index and obesity in the United States, 1971-2002. *Archives of Internal Medicine, 165*(18), 2122-8; Wang Y., Zhang Q. (2006). Are American children and adolescents of low socioeconomic status at increased risk of obesity?: Changes in the association between overweight and family income between 1971-2002. *American Journal of Clinical Nutrition, 84*(4), 707-16.

[22] Wang Y., Zhang Q. (2006). Are American children and adolescents of low socioeconomic status at increased risk of obesity?: Changes in the association between overweight and family income between 1971-2002. *American Journal of Clinical Nutrition, 84*(4), 707-16.

[23] Centers for Disease Control and Prevention. (n.d.) Obesity Trends: Trends by State 1985-2008. Retrieved March 7, 2010 from: http://www.cdc.gov/obesity

[24] Pleis J.R., Lucas J.W., Ward B.W. (2009). Summary health statistics for U.S. dults: National Health Interview Survey, 2008. *Vital and Health Statistics. Series, 10*(242). Washington, D.C.: Government Printing Office.

[25] Expert Panel on the Identification, Evaluation, and Treatment of Overweight in Adults. (1998). Clinical guidelines on the identification, evaluation, and treatment of overweight and obesity in adults: executive summary. *American Journal of Clinical Nutrition, 68*(4), 899-917.

[26] Singh A.S., Mulder C., Twisk J.W., et al. (2008). Tracking of childhood overweight into adulthood: a systematic review of the literature. *Obesity Reviews, 9*(5), 474-88; Freedman D., Wang J., Thornton J.C., et al. (2009). Classification of body fatness by body mass index-for-age categories among children. *Archives of Pediatrics & Adolescent Medicine,163*(9), 805-11; Flegal K.M., Shepherd J.A., Looker A.C., et al. (2009). Comparisons of percentage body fat, body mass index, waist circumference, and waist-stature ratio in adults. *American Journal of Clinical Nutrition, 89*(2), 500-508.

[27] Freedman, D.S., Khan, L.K., Serdula, M.K., et al. (2005). The relation of childhood BMI to adult adiposity: the Bogalusa Heart Study. *Pediatrics, 115*(1), 22-7.

[28] Whitlock, E.P., Williams, S.B., Gold, R., et al. (2005). Screening and interventions for childhood overweight: a summary of evidence for the US Preventive Services Task Force. *Pediatrics, 116*(1), el 25-44.

[29] Daniels, S.R., Arnett, D.K., Eckel, R.H., et al. (2005). Overweight in children and adolescents: pathophysiology, consequences, prevention, and treatment. *Circulation, 111*(15), 1999-2012.

[30] Freedman, D.S., Mei, Z., Srinivasan, S.R., et al. (2007). Cardiovascular risk factors and excess adiposity among overweight children and adolescents: the Bogalusa Heart Study. *Journal of Pediatrics 150*(1), 12-17 e2.

[31] Kaevey, R.E., Daniels et al. (2007). Cardiovascular Risk Reduction in High-Risk Pediatric Patients. *Journal of Cardiovascular Nursing 22*(3), 218-53.

[32] Berenson, G.S., Srinivasan, S.R., Bao, W., et al. (1998). Association between multiple cardiovascular risk factors and atherosclerosis in children and young adults: the Bogalusa Heart Study. *New England Journal of Medicine, 338*(23), 1650-6.

[33] Gilliland, F.D., Berhane, K., Islam, T., et al. (2003). Obesity and the risk of newly diagnosed asthma in school-age children. *American Journal of Epidemiology, 158*(5), 406-15.

[34] Lee, J.M., Okumura, M.J., Freed, G.L., et al. (2007). Trends in hospitalizations for diabetes among children and young adults: United States, 1993-2004. *Diabetes Care, 30*(12), 3035-9.

[35] Mayer-Davis, E.J., Bell, R.A., Dabelea, D., et al. (2009). The many faces of diabetes in American youth: type 1 and type 2 diabetes in five race and ethnic populations: the SEARCH for Diabetes in Youth Study. *Diabetes Care, 32*(Supplemental 2), S99-101.

[36] Cogswell, M.E., Scanlon, K.S., Fein, S.B., Schieve, L.A. (1999). Medically advised, mother's personal target, and actual weight gain during pregnancy. *Obstetrics & Gynecology, 94*(4), 616-622.

[37] Schwimmer, J.B, Burwinkle, T.M., Varni, J.W. (2003). Health-Related Quality of Life of Severely Obese Children and Adolescents. *Journal of the American Medical Association, 289*, 1813-1819.

[38] Strauss R.S. (2000). Childhood obesity and self-esteem. *Pediatrics, 105*(1), e15.

[39] Rofey et al. (2009). A longitudinal study of childhood depression and anxiety in relation to weight gain. *Child Psychiatry and Human Development, 40*, 517-526; Tanofsky-Kraff et al. (2006). A prospective study of psychological predictors of body fat gain among children at high risk for adult obesity. *Pediatrics, 117*(4), 1203-9.

[40] Gillman M.W. (2008a). The first months of life: a critical period for development of obesity. *American Journal of Clinical Nutrition, 87*(6), 1587-9.

[41] Fisher D., Baird J., Payne L., et al. (2006). Are infant size and growth related to burden of disease in adulthood? A systematic review of literature. *International Journal of Epidemiology, 35*(5), 1196-210.

[42] Gillman M.W. (2008a). The first months of life: a critical period for development of obesity. *American Journal of Clinical Nutrition, 87*(6), 1587-9; Gillman M.W., Rifas-Shiman S.L., Kleinman K., et al. (2008b). Developmental origins of childhood overweight: potential public health impact. *Obesity, 16*(7), 1651-6; Gardner D.S., Hosking J., Metcalf B.S., et al. (2009). Contribution of early weight gain to childhood overweight and metabolic health: a longitudinal study (Early Bird 36). *Pediatrics, 123*(1), e67-73.

[43] Taveras E.M., Gillman M.W., Kleinman K., et al. (2010). Racial/Ethnic differences in early-life risk factors for childhood obesity. *Pediatrics, 125*(4), 686-95; Stunkard A.J., Harris J.R., Pedersen N.L., McClearn G.E. (1990). The body mass index of twins who have been reared apart. *New England Journal of Medicine, 322*, 1483–1487; Han J.C., Liu Q.R., Jones M., Levinn R.L., Menzie C.M., Jefferson-George K.S., Adler-Wailes D.C., Sanford E.L., Lacbawan F.L., Uhl G.R., Rennert O.M., Yanovski J.A. (2008). Brain-Derived Neurotrophic Factor and Obesity in the WAGR Syndrome. *New England Journal of Medicine, 359*, 918.

[44] Maes H., Neale M.C., Eaves L.J. (1997). Genetic and environmental factors in relative body weight and human obesity. *Behavior Genetics, 27*, 325–351.

[45] Stunkar A.J., Harris J.R., Pedersen N.L., McClearn G.E. (1990). The body-mass index of twins who have been reared apart. *New England Journal of Medicine, 322*, 1483-87.

[46] O'Rahilly S. and Farooqi I.S. (2008). Human obesity: a heritable neurobehavioral disorder that is highly sensitive to environmental conditions. *Diabetes, 57*, 2905-10.

[47] Guthrie J.F., Lin B.H., Frazao E. (2002). Role of food prepared away from home in the American diet, 1977-78 versus 1994-96: changes and consequences. *Journal of Nutrition Education and Behavior, 34*(3), 140-50.

[48] Federal Trade Commission (2008). *Marketing food to children and adolescents: a review of industry expenditure, activities, and self-regulation. A Federal Trade Commission Report to Congress.* Washington, D.C.: Federal Trade Commission.

[49] Wang Y.C., Bleich S.N., Gortmaker S.L. (2008). Increasing caloric contribution from sugar-sweetened beverages and 100% fruit juices among U.S. children and adolescents, 1988-2004. *Pediatrics, 121*(6), e1 604-14.

[50] McDonald N.C. (2007). Active transportation to school: trends among U.S. schoolchildren, 1969-2001. *American Journal of Preventive Medicine, 32*(6), 509-1 6.

[51] McDonald N.C. (2007). Active transportation to school: trends among U.S. schoolchildren, 1969-2001. *American Journal of Preventive Medicine, 32*(6), 509-1 6.

[52] Dietz W.H., Gortmaker S.L. (2001). Preventing obesity in children and adolescents. *Annual Review of Public Health, 22*, 337-53.

[53] Taveras E.M., Sandora T.J., Shih M-C., Ross-Degnan D., Goldmann D.A., Gillman M.W. (2006). The association of television and video viewing with fast food intake by preschool age children. *Obesity, 14*, 2034- 41; Harris, J.L., Bargh J.A., Brownell, K.D. (2009). Priming effects of television advertising on eating behavior. *Health Psychology 28*(4), 404–413.

[54] Owens, J.A. (2010). Sleep: The Missing Link in Preventing Childhood Obesity. Warren Alpert Medical School of Brown University; Quan, S.F., Parthasarathy, S., Budhiraga, R. (2010). Healthy Sleep Education—A Salve for Obesity? *Journal of Clinical Sleep Medicine, 6*(1), 18-19.

[55] Anderson, S., Whitaker, R. (2010). Household routines and obesity in U.S. Pre-school-Aged Children. Pediatrics, 125(3), 420-428; Taveras, E.M., Rifas-Shiman, S., et al. (2008). Short sleep duration in infancy and risk of childhood overweight. *Archives of Pediatrics & Adolescent Medicine, 162(4)*, 305-311.

[56] Centers for Disease Control and Prevention. (2009). Recommended Community Strategies and Measurements to Prevent Obesity in the United States. *Morbidity and Mortality Weekly Report, July 24, 2009.* Retrieved from: http://www.cdc.gov/mmwr/preview/mmwrhtml/rr5807a1.htm.

[57] Robert Wood Johnson Foundation (2009). *Healthy Kids, Healthy Communities: Supporting Community Action to Prevent Childhood Obesity.* Retrieved from: http://www.healthykidshealthycommunities.org/.

[58] The California Endowment (2010). *First Lady Michelle Obama comes to California to announce the official launch of The California Endowment's Building Healthy Communities Initiative in partnership with her Let's Move! campaign.* Retrieved from: http://www.calendow.org/Article.aspx?id=4415.

[59] Haby, M.M., Vos, T., Carter, R., Moodie, M., Markwick, A., Magnus, A., et al. (2006). A new approach to assessing the health benefit from obesity interventions in children and adolescents: the assessing cost-effectiveness in obesity project. *International Journal of Obesity, 30*(10), 1463-75; Roux, L., Pratt, M., Tengs, T.O., Yore, M.M., Yanagawa, T.L., Van Den Bos, J., et al. (2008). Cost effectiveness of community-based physical activity interventions. *American Journal of Preventive Medicine, 35*(6), 578-88.

[60] Fungwe, T., Guenther, P.M. Juan, W. Hiza, H.,Lino, M. (2009). The Quality of Children's Diets in 2003-04 as Measured by the Healthy Eating Index-2005. *Nutrition Insight, 43.* Alexandria, V.A.: U.S. Department of Agriculture, Center for Nutrition Policy and Promotion.

[61] Ogden C.L., Carroll M.D., Curtin LR, et al. (2010). Prevalence of high body mass index in US children and adolescents, 2007-2008. *Journal of the American Medical Association 303*(3), 242-9.

[62] Harrington, J.W. et a l., (2010). Identifying the Tipping Point Age for Overweight Pediatric Patients, *Clinical Pediatrics, 49*(3).

[63] Kim, J., Peterson, K. E., Scanlon, K. S., Fitzmaurice, G. M., Must, A., Oken, E., Rifas-Shiman, S. L., Rich-Edwards, J. W., and Gillman, M. W. (2006). Trends in overweight from 1980 through 2001 among preschool-aged children enrolled in a health maintenance organization. *Obesity, 14,* 1107-12.

[64] Committee on the Impact of Pregnancy Weight on Maternal and Child Health. (2007). *National Research Council Influence of Pregnancy Weight on Maternal and Child Health: Workshop Report.* Washington, DC: The National Academies Press.

[65] Wells, J., Chomtho S., Fewtrell, M. (2007). Programming of body composition by early growth and nutrition. *Proceedings of the Nutrition Society,* 423-434.

[66] Committee on the Impact of Pregnancy Weight on Maternal and Child Health. (2007). *National Research Council Influence of Pregnancy Weight on Maternal and Child Health: Workshop Report.* Washington, DC: The National Academies Press.

[67] Kohta, S. et al. (2009). The Association between Maternal Smoking during Pregnancy and Childhood Obesity Persists to the Age of 9–10 Years. *Journal of Epidemiology, 19,* 136-142.

[68] Sharma A.J., et al. (2008). Dose-Response Associations Between Maternal Smoking During Pregnancy and Subsequent Childhood Obesity: Effect Modification by Maternal Race/Ethnicity in a Low-Income U.S. *American Journal of Epidemiology, 168,* 995-1007.

[69] Section 4107 ("Coverage of Comprehensive Tobacco Cessation Services for Pregnant Women in Medicaid") of the Patient Protection and Affordable Care Act of 2010, Pub. L. No 111-148.

[70] U.S. Department of Health and Human Services. (2010). *The Surgeon General's Vision for a Healthy and Fit Nation.* Retrieved from: http://www.surgeongeneral.gov/library/obesityvision/obesityvision.pdf.

[71] Wolff S., Legarth J., Vangsgaard K., Toubro S., Astrup A. (2008). A randomized trial of the effects of dietary counseling on gestational weight gain and glucose metabolism in obese pregnant women. *International Journal of Obesity, 32*(3), 495-501; Asbee S.M., Jenkins T.R., Butler J.R., White J., Elliot M., Rutledge A. (2009). Preventing excessive weight gain during pregnancy through dietary and lifestyle counseling: a randomized controlled trial. *Obstetrics & Gynecology, 113*(2 Pt 1), 305-12.

[72] Cogswell M.E., Scanlon K.S., Fein S.B., Schieve L.A. (1999). Medically advised, mother's personal target, and actual weight gain during pregnancy. *Obstetrics & Gynecology, 94*(4), 616-22; Stotland N.E., Haas J.S., Brawarsky P., Jackson R.A., Fuentes-Afflick E., Escobar G.J. (2005). Body mass index, provider advice, and target gestational weight gain. *Obstetrics & Gynecology, 105*(3), 633-8.

[73] Institute of Medicine. (2009). *Weight Gain During Pregnancy: Reexamining the Guidelines.* Washington, DC: The National Academies Press; Gunderson E.P. (2009). Childbearing and obesity in women: weight before, during, and after pregnancy. *Obstetrics & Gynecology Clinics of North America, 36*(2), 317-32, ix; Rooney B.L., Schauberger C.W., Mathiason M.A. (2005). Impact of perinatal weight change on long-term obesity and obesity-related illnesses. *Obstetrics & Gynecology, 106*(6),1 349-56.

[74] Institute of Medicine. (2009). *Weight Gain During Pregnancy: Reexamining the Guidelines.* Washington, DC: The National Academies Press.

[75] Centers for Disease Control and Prevention , National Vital Statistics System. (2003). 2003 Revisions of the U.S. Standard Certificates of Live Birth and Death and the Fetal Death Report, and U.S. Standard Certificate of Live Birth. Retrieved on April 8, 2010 from http://www.cdc.gov/nchs/nvss/vital_certificate and http://www.cdc.gov/nchs/data/dvs/birth11-03final-ACC.pdf.

[76] Hamilton B.E., Martin J.A., Ventura S.J.. Births: Preliminary data for 2007. *National vital statistics reports,* 57(12) Retrieved from: http://www.cdc.gov/nchs/data/nvsr/nvsr57/nvsr57_12.pdf.

[77] Owen C.G., Martin R.M., Whincup P.H., Davey Smith G., Cook D.G. (2005). Effect of infant feeding on the risk of obesity across the life course: a quantitative review of the published evidence. *Pediatrics, 115,* 1367-1377.

[78] Arenz S., Ruckerl R., Koletzko B., Von Kries R. (2004). Breast-feeding and childhood obesity: a systematic review. *International Journal of Obesity and Related Metabolic Disorders, 28,* 1247-1256.

[79] Harder T., Bergmann R., Kallischnigg G., Plagemann A.. (2005). Duration of breastfeeding and risk of overweight: a meta-analysis. *American Journal of Epidemiology, 162,* 397-403.

[80] Centers for Disease Control and Prevention, Division of Nutrition, Physical Activity and Obesity, National Center for Chronic Disease Prevention and Health Promotion. (2006). Breastfeeding Among U.S. Children Born 1999—2006, CDC National Immunization Survey. Retrieved from http://www.cdc.gov/breastfeeding

[81] Scanlon K.S., Grummer-Strawn L., Li R., Chen J., Molinari N., Perrine C.G. (2010). Racial and ethnic differences in breastfeeding initiation and duration, by state – National Immunization Survey, U.S., 2004-2008. *Morbidity and Mortality Weekly Report, 59*(11), 327-334.

[82] Heinig M.J., Nommsen L.A., Peerson J.M., et al. (1993). Energy and protein intakes of breast-fed and formula-fed infants during the first year of life and their association with growth velocity: the DARLING Study. *American Journal of Clinical Nutrition, 58,* 152-161.

[83] Hondares E., Rosell M., Gonzales F., Giralt M., Iglesias, Villarroya F. (2010). Hepatic FGF21 expression is induced at birth via PPARα in response to milk intake and contributes to thermogenic activation of neonatal brown fat. *Cell Metabolism , 11,* 206-212.

[84] Lucas A., Boyes S., Bloom R., Aynsley-Green A.. (1981). Metabolic and endocrine responses to a milk feed in six-day-old term infants: differences between breast and cow's milk formula feeding. *Acta paediatrica Scandinavica, 70,* 195-200.

[85] Singhal A., Farooqi I.S., O'Rahilly S., et al. (2002). Early nutrition and leptin concentrations in later life. *American Journal of Clinical Nutrition, 75,* 993-999.
[86] Centers for Disease Control and Prevention, Division of Nutrition, Physical Activity and Obesity, National Center for Chronic Disease Prevention and Health Promotion. (2008). Infant Feeding Practices Study II. *Pediatrics, 122* (Special Issue Supplement).
[87] Centers for Disease Control and Prevention. (2009). Breastfeeding Report Card – United States, Retrieved from: http://www.cdc.gov/breastfeeding
[88] Kramer, M.S. (1981). Do breast-feeding and delayed introduction of solid foods protect against subsequent obesity? *Journal of Pediatrics 98,* 883-87; Wilson, A,C,, Forsyth J,S,, Greene S,A,, Irvine L,, Hau C,, Howie P,W, (1998). Relation of infant diet to childhood health: seven year follow up of cohorot of children in Dundee infant study. *British Medical Journal 316,* 21 -25; Taveras, E., Gillman, E., Gillman, M., Kleinman, K., Rich- Edwards, J, Rifas-Shiman, S. (2010). Racial/Ethnic Differences in Early-Life Risk Factors for Childhood Obesity. *Pediatrics, 125* (4), 686-95.
[89] U.S. States Breastfeeding Committee. (2002). *Breastfeeding and child care* [Issue paper]. Raleigh, NC: United States Breastfeeding Committee. Retrieved from: http://www.usbreastfeeding.org/Portals/0/Publications/Child%20Care-2002-USBC.pdf
[90] Society for Human Resource Management. (2009). 2009 Employee Benefits: Examining Employee Benefits in a Fiscally Challenging Economy. Retrieved from: http://www.shrm.org/Research/SurveyFindings/Articles/Documents/09-0295_Employee_Benefits_Survey_Report_spread_FNL.pdf.
[91] Section 4207 ("Reasonable Break Time for Nursing Mothers") of the Patient Protection and Affordable Care Act of 2010, Pub. L. No 111-148.
[92] U.S. Department of Health and Human Services, Health Resources and Services Administration (HRSA), Maternal and Child Health Bureau (2008). The Business Case for Breastfeeding [Video file]. Retrieved from: http://webcast.hrsa.gov/postevents/archivedWebcastDetailNewInterface.asp?aeid=454.
[93] Batan MC, Li R, Scanlon KSS. (2010, November). Is child care providers' support for breastfeeding associated with breastfeeding duration? Abstract submitted for presentation at American Public Health Association 138th Annual Meeting and Expo.
[94] Kistin N., Benton, D., Rao S., Sullivan, M. (1990). Breast-Feeding Rates Among Black Urban Low-Income Women: Effect of Prenatal Education. *Pediatrics, 86*(5), 741-746.
[95] Chung M., Raman G., Trikalinos T., Lau J., Ip S. (2008). Interventions in primary care to promote breastfeeding: an evidence review for the U.S. Preventive Services Task Force. *Annals of Internal Medicine, 149*(8), 565 - 82.
[96] Section 2951 ("Maternal, Infant, and Early Childhood Home Visitation Programs") of the Patient Protection and Affordable Care Act of 2010, Pub. L. no 111-148.
[97] Examples of these chemicals include several estrogenic chemicals (e.g. genistein, diethylstilbestrol, bisphenol A), perfluorooctanoic acid (PFOA), smoking/nicotine, tributyltin, phthalates, fructose, monosodium glutamate, and certain organophosphate pesticides. In addition, other environmental chemicals have been associated with diabetes in humans, including arsenic, cadmium, dioxin, polychlorinated biphenyls (PCBs) and other types of halogenated organic compounds. Longnecker, M. P., and Daniels, J. L. (2001). Environmental contaminants as etiologic factors for diabetes. *Environmental Health Perspectives, 109*(Supplemental 6), 871-6; Edwards, J. R., and Prozialeck, W. C. (2009). Cadmium, diabetes and chronic kidney disease. *Toxicology and Applied Pharmacology, 238*, 289-93; Schwartz, G. G., Il'yasova, D., and Ivanova, A. (2003). Urinary cadmium, impaired fasting glucose, and diabetes in the NHANES III. Diabetes Care, 26, 468-70; Tseng, C. H. (2004). The potential biological mechanisms of arsenic-induced diabetes mellitus. Toxicology and Applied Pharmacology, 197, 67-83; Turyk, M., Anderson, H. A.,Knobeloch, L., Imm, P., and Persky, V. W. (2009). Prevalence of diabetes and body burdens of polychlorinated biphenyls, polybrominated diphenyl ethers, and p,p'-diphenyldichloroethene in Great Lakes sport fish consumers. *Chemosphere, 75*, 674-9; Uemura, H., Arisawa, K., Hiyoshi, M., Kitayama, A., Takami, H., Sawachika, F., Dakeshita, S., Nii, K., Satoh, H., Sumiyoshi, Y., Morinaga, K., Kodama, K., Suzuki, T., Nagai, M., and Suzuki, T. (2009). Prevalence of metabolic syndrome associated with body burden levels of dioxin and related compounds among Japan's general population. Environmental Health Perspectives, 117, 568-73; Grun, F. and B. Blumberg, Endocrine disrupters as obesogens. Mol Cell Endocrinol, 2009. 304(1-2): p. 19-29.
[98] U.S. Department of Health and Human Services. (n.d.) Bisphenol A (BPA) Information for Parents. Retrieved from: http://www.hhs.gov/safety
[99] American Academy of Pediatrics Committee on Public Education. (2001). Children, Adolescents, and Television. Retrieved from: http://aappolicy.aappublications.org/cgi/reprint/pediatrics;107/2/423.pdf.
[100] Rideout V., Vandewater E., Wartel la, E. (2003). *Zero to Six: Electronic Media in the Lives of Infants, Toddlers and Preschoolers.* Menlo Park, C.A.: Henry J. Kaiser Foundation.

[101] Rideout, V., Hame, E. (2006). *The Media Family: Electronic Media in the Lives of Infants, Toddlers, Preschoolers and Their Parents.* Menlo Park, C.A.: Henry J. Kaiser Family Foundation. Retrieved from: http://www.kff.org/entmedia/upload/7500.pdf

[102] Dennison, B.A., Erb, T.A., & Jenkins, P.L. (2002). Television viewing and television in bedroom associated with overweight risk among low-income preschool children. *Pediatrics, 109*, 1028–1035.

[103] Mendoza J.A., Zimmerman F.J., Christakis D.A.. (2007). Television viewing and obesity in U.S. preschool children. *International Journal of Behavioral Nutrition and Physical Activity, 4*(1), 44.

[104] Taveras, E.M., Sandora, T.J., Shihm, M.C., Ross-Degnan, D., Goldmann, D.A., Gillman M.W. (2006). The association of television and video viewing with fast food intake by preschool-age children. *Obesity (Silver Spring), 14*(11), 2034-41.

[105] U.S. Census Bureau. (2005). Survey of Program Participation: Child Care. Retrieved from: http://www.census.gov/population

[106] U.S. Census Bureau Survey of Income and Program Participation, Spring 2005, unpublished data.

[107] Whitaker, R. C., Pepe, M. S., Knight, J. A., Seidel, K. D., & Dietz, W. H. (1998). Early adiposity rebound and the risk of adult obesity. *Pediatrics, 101*(3), 5; Maher, E.J., Li, G., Carter L., Johnson D.B. (2008). Preschool child care participation and obesity at the start of kindergarten. *Pediatrics, 122*(2), 322-30.

[108] McWilliams C., et al. (2009). Best Practice Guidelines for PA in Child Care. Pediatrics,1 24(6), 1650-1659; Hannon, J.C., Brown B.B. (2008). Increasing preschoolers' physical activity intensities: an activity-friendly preschool playground intervention. *Preventative Medicine, 46*(6); Dowda, M., Brown, W.H., McIver, K.L., et al. (2009). Policies and characteristics of the preschool environment and physical activity of young children. *Pediatrics, 123,* 261-266.

[109] Bruening K.S., Gilbride J.A., Passannante M.R., McClowry S. (1999). Dietary intake and health outcomes among young children attending 2 urban day-care centers. *Journal of the American Dietetic Association, 99*(12), 1529-35.

[110] Chandran, K. (2009, September). Improving Nutrition in Child Care in America. Presentation for the Nemours *Healthy Kids, Healthy Future Convening.* Washington, DC.

[111] Kaphingst, K.M., Story, M. (2009). Child Care as Untapped Setting for Obesity Prevention. *Prevention Chronic Disease, 6*(1).

[112] Benjamin, S.E., Finkelstein, J. (2010). Preventing Obesity in the Child Care Setting: Evaluating State Regulations. Retrieved from: http://cfm.mc.duke.edu/modules

[113] *Caring for our Children: National Health and Safety Performance Standards* is published by the National Resource Center for Health and Safety in Child Care and Early Education. The National Resource Center is funded by the Maternal and Child Health Bureau, U.S. Department of Health & Human Services, HRSA.

[114] Lin BH, Guthrie J, Frazao E. (2001). American children's diets not making the grade. *Food Review, 24*(2), 8-17; Center for Disease Control and Prevention. (2008). Youth Risk Behavior Surveillance—United States, 2007. Morbidity & Mortality Weekly Report, 57(SS-05), 1–131.

[115] Bittman, M. (2009). *Food Matters: A Guide to Conscious Eating.* New York, NY: Simon & Schuster; Pollan, M. (2009). *Food Rules: An Eater's Manual.* New York, NY: Penguin Books; Heath, C., Heath, D. (2010). *Switch: How to Change Things When Change is Hard.* New York, NY: Random House.

[116] Section 4004 ("Education and Outreach Campaign Regarding Preventive Benefits") of the Patient Protection and Affordable Care Act of 2010, Pub. L. No 111-148.

[117] U.S. Department of Agriculture, Food Safety and Inspection Service. (2009). Nutrition Labeling of Single-Ingredient Products and Ground or Chopped Meat and Poultry Products: Proposed Rule. *Federal Register, 74*(242), 67735-67800.

[118] U.S. Health and Human Services, Food and Drug Administration. (2010). *Key Findings from 2002 and 2008 U.S Food and Drug Administration's Health and Diet Survey.* [Facts heet]. Retrieved from: www.fda.gov/Food/LabelingNutrition/ucm202780.htm

[119] Choinière, C.J., Lando, A. (2008). 2008 Health and Diet Survey. Retrieved from: http://www.fda.gov/Food/ScienceResearch/ResearchAreas/ConsumerResearch/ucm193895.htm

[120] On March 3, 2010, FDA Commissioner issued an open letter to industry on the importance of accurate nutrition labeling of food products, and the agency issued Warning Letters to 17 manufacturers informing the firms that the labeling for 22 of their food products violate provisions of the Federal Food, Drug, and Cosmetic Act that require labels to be truthful and not misleading.

[121] Section 4205 ("Nutrition labeling of standard menu items at chain restaurants") of the Patient Protection and Affordable Care Act of 2010, Pub. L. No 111-148.

[122] Nestle, M. (2010). Health Care Reform in Action—Calorie Labeling Goes National. *New England Journal of Medicine.* Retrieved from: http://www.NEJM.org

[123] Wisdom, J., Downs, J.S., Loewenstein, G. (2010). Promoting Healthy Choices: Information versus Convenience. *American Economic Journal: Applied Economics, 2,* 164–178.

[124] Wansink, B., Just, D.R., Payne, C.R. (2009). Mindless Eating and Healthy Heuristics for the Irrational. *American Economic Review: Papers & Proceedings, 99*(2), 165–169.

[125] Wansink, B., Kim J. (2005). Bad Popcorn in Big Buckets: Portion Size Can Influence Intake as Much as Taste. *Journal of Nutrition Education and Behavior, 37*(5), 242-5.

[126] Nielsen, S.J., Popkin, B.M. (2003). Patterns and trends in food portion sizes, 1977-1998. *Journal of the American Medical Association, 289*(4), 450-453.

[127] Anderson, S., Whitaker, R. (2010). Household routines and obesity in U.S. Pre-school-Aged Children. *Pediatrics, 125*(3), 420-428; Taveras, E.M., Rifas-Shiman, S., et al. (2008). Short sleep duration in infancy and risk of childhood overweight. Archives of Pediatrics & Adolescent Medicine, 162(4), 305 311.

[128] Anderson, S., Whitaker, R. (2010). Household routines and obesity in U.S. Pre-school-Aged Children. *Pediatrics, 125*(3), 420-428; Taveras, E.M., Rifas-Shiman, S., et al. (2008). Short sleep duration in infancy and risk of childhood overweight. Archives of Pediatrics & Adolescent Medicine, 162(4), 900-906.

[129] U.S. General Accounting Office. (2004). *Nutrition Education: USDA Provides Services through Multiple Programs, but Stronger Linkages among Efforts Are Needed.* Washington, D.C.: U.S. General Accounting Office.

[130] Economic Research Service (ERS), U.S. Department of Agriculture (USDA). (1997). Understanding Food Prices. *Food Review, 20*(2).

[131] Federal Trade Commission. (2008) *Marketing Food to Children and Adolescents: A Review of Industry Expenditures, Activities, and Self-Regulation.* Washington, D.C.: Federal Trade Commission. Retrieved from: http://www.ftc.gov/os/2008/07/P064504foodmktingreport.pdf, at ES-1.

[132] Escobar-Chaves, S.L., Anderson, C.A. (2008). Media and Risky Behaviors. Children and Electronic Media. 18(1).Retrieved from: http://futureofchildren.org/futureofchildren/publications/docs/18_01_07.pdf

[133] Institute Of Medicine. Committee on Food Marketing and the Diets of Children and Youth. (2006). *Food Marketing to Children and Youth, Threat or Opportunity?* Washington, D.C.: The National Academies Press.

[134] Institute Of Medicine. Committee on *Food Marketing and the Diets of Children and Youth. (2006). Food Marketing to Children and Youth, Threat or Opportunity?* Washington, D.C.; The National Academies Press; Gantz, W. et al. (2007). Food for Thought, Television Advertising to Children in the United States. Menlo Park, C.A.: The Henry Kaiser Family Foundation.

[135] Robinson T.N., Borzekowski D.L.G., Matheson D.M., Kraimer H.C. (2007). Effects of fast food branding on young children's taste preferences. *Archives of Pediatrics & Adolescent Medicine, 161,* 792-797.

[136] Federal Trade Commission. (2008). *Marketing Food to Children and Adolescents: A Review of Industry Expenditures, Activities, and Self-Regulation.* Washington, D.C.: Federal Trade Commission. Retrieved from: http://www.ftc.gov/os/2008/07/P064504foodmktingreport.pdf, at ES-2, 8.

[137] Federal Trade Commission. (2008). *Marketing Food to Children and Adolescents: A Review of Industry Expenditures, Activities, and Self-Regulation.* Washington, D.C.: Federal Trade Commission. Retrieved from: http://www.ftc.gov/os/2008/07/P064504foodmktingreport.pdf, ES 4-6.

[138] Federal Trade Commission. (2008). *Marketing Food to Children and Adolescents: A Review of Industry Expenditures, Activities, and Self-Regulation.* Washington, D.C.: Federal Trade Commission. Retrieved from http://www.ftc.gov/os/2008/07/P064504foodmktingreport.pdf, ES-4.

[139] Sesame Workshop. (2005, September 20). *The Effectiveness of Characters on Children's Food Choices* [Press Release]. Retrieved at: http://archive.sesameworkshop.org/aboutus/inside_press.php?contentId=15092302.

[140] Harris, J., et al. (2009). Marketing Foods to Children and Adolescents: Licensed Characters and Other Promotions on Packaged Foods in the Supermarket. *Public Health Nutrition, 13*(3), 409-417. This recent study by the Yale University Rudd Center for Food Policy and Obesity found a substantial increase (78%) in the number of food products with youth-oriented cross-promotions on packaging between 2006 and 2008. Nearly 75% of those cross-promotions involved the use of licensed characters.

[141] Harris, J., et al. (2009). Marketing Foods to Children and Adolescents: Licensed Characters and Other Promotions on Packaged Foods in the Supermarket. *Public Health Nutrition, 13*(3), 409-417.

[142] Children's Food and Beverage Advertising Initiative. (n.d.). Retrieved from: http://www.bbb.org/us/children

[143] Effective January 1, 2010, this principle was expanded to apply to advertising through video games and cell phones, as well as word-of-mouth advertising. Children's Food and Beverage Advertising Initiative. (n.d.). Retrieved from http://www.bbb.org/us/enhanced-core-principles

[144] Federal Trade Commission. (2008). *Marketing Food to Children and Adolescents: A Review of Industry Expenditures, Activities, and Self-Regulation.* Washington, D.C.: Federal Trade Commission. Retrieved from: http://www.ftc.gov/os/2008/07/P064504foodmktingreport.pdf, 63-64.

[145] Federal Trade Commission. (2008) *Marketing Food to Children and Adolescents: A Review of Industry Expenditures, Activities, and Self-Regulation.* Washington, D.C.: Federal Trade Commission. Retrieved from: http://www.ftc.gov/os/2008/07/P064504foodmktingreport.pdf, 64-65.

[146] Kunkel, D. et al. (2009). *The Impact of Industry Self-Regulation on the Nutritional Quality of Foods Advertised on Television to Children.* Retrieved from: http://www.childrennow.org/uploads/documents/adstudy_2009.pdf.

[147] Kunkel, D. et al. (2009). *The Impact of Industry Self-Regulation on the Nutritional Quality of Foods Advertised on Television to Children.* Retrieved from: http://www.childrennow.org/uploads/documents/adstudy_2009.pdf

[148] Kunkel, D. et al. (2009). *The Impact of Industry Self-Regulation on the Nutritional Quality of Foods Advertised on Television to Children.* Retrieved from: http://www.childrennow.org/uploads/documents/adstudy_2009.pdf

[149] Letter from Maureen Enright, Assistant Director, CFBAI, and Elaine D. Kolish, Vice President and Director, CFBAI, to Marlene H. Dortch, Secretary, FCC, dated March 26, 2010, in MB Docket 09-194.

[150] For example, the Walt Disney Company, Nickelodeon, Cartoon Network, and Sesame Workshop.

[151] Federal Trade Commission Report to Congress. (2008). *Marketing Food to Children and Adolescents: A Review of Industry, Expenditures, Activities and Self-Regulation.* Retrieved from: http://www.ftc.gov/os/2008/07/P064504foodmktingreport.pdf

[152] U.S. House. Appropriations Committee.(2009). Division D – Financial Services and General Government, Explanatory Statement, Title V, Independent Agencies, 983-84. Retrieved from: http://frwebgate.access dbname=1 1 1_cong_house_committee_prints&docid=f:47494d.pdf

[153] Kunkel, D. et al. (2009). *The Impact of Industry Self-Regulation on the Nutritional Quality of Foods Advertised on Television to Children.* Retrieved from: http://www.childrennow.org/uploads/documents/adstudy_2009.pdf.

[154] Section 303 ("Standards for children's television programming") of the Children's Television Act of 1990, Pub. L. 101-437.

[155] FTC has played an important role in addressing issues of food marketing, childhood nutrition, and obesity. Since 2005, it has hosted three public workshops and issued two reports, including its landmark 2008 report to Congress: *Marketing Food to Children and Adolescents: A Review of Industry Expenditures, Activities, and Self-Regulation.* FTC is currently preparing to conduct a follow up study, expected to be published in 2011, and is participating in the IWG to develop recommendations for voluntary uniform nutritional standards for child-directed food and beverage marketing.

[156] Holt, D., Ippolito, P., Desrochers, D., Kelley, C. (2007). *Children's Exposure to TV Advertising in 1977 and 2004.* Washington, D.C.: Federal Trade Commission, Bureau of Economics Staff Report. ES-7-8. Retrieved from: http://www.ftc.gov/os/2007/06/cabebw.pdf

[157] On average, more than 3 million children watched American Idol in 2005-2006 and more than 1 million watched *The Simpsons.* By comparison, the average child audience for SpongeBob Square Pants was 2 million. Federal Trade Commission. (2008). *Marketing Food to Children and Adolescents: A Review of Industry Expenditures, Activities, and Self-Regulation.* Washington, D.C.: Federal Trade Commission. Retrieved from: http://www.ftc.gov/os/2008/07/P064504foodmktingreport.pdf, 15-16.

[158] Doolen, J., Alpert, P.T., Miller, S.K. (2009). Parental disconnect between perceived and actual weight status of children: a metasynthesis of the current research. *Journal of the American Academy of Nurse Practitioners, 21*(3), 160-6.

[159] National health objectives can be found in Healthy People 2010. Overweight and Obesity. (n.d.) Retrieved October 15, 2009 from: http://www.healthypeople.gov/Document/html/uih/uih_bw/uih_4.htm#overandobese.

[160] Freedman D., Wang J., Thornton J.C., et al. (2009). Classification of body fatness by body mass indexfor-age categories among children. *Archives of Pediatrics & Adolescent Medicine, 163*(9), 805-11.

[161] Klein, J.D., Sesselberg, T.S., Johnson, M.S., O'Connor, K.G., Cook, S., Coon, M., Homer, C., Krebs, N., Washington, R. (2010). Adoption of body mass index guidelines for screening and counseling in pediatric practice. Pediatrics, 125(2), 265-72.

[162] Centers for Disease Control and Prevention. (2005). Children and teens told by doctors that they were overweight, United States, 1999-2002. *Morbidity and Mortality Weekly Report, 54*(34), 848-9.

[163] Nihiser, A.J., Lee, S.M., Wechsler, H., McKenna, M,, Odom, E., Reinold, C., Thompson, D., GrummerStrawn, L. (2007). Body mass index measurement in schools. *Journal of School Health. 77*(10), 651-71; Nihiser, A.J., Lee, S.M., Wechsler, H., McKenna, M,, Odom, E., Reinold, C., Thompson, D., Grummer-Strawn, L. (2007). Body mass index measurement in schools. *Journal of School Health. 77*(Supplemental 1), S89-97.

[164] U.S. Department of Health and Human Services. (2010). *The Surgeon General's Vision for a Healthy and Fit Nation.* Rockville, MD: U.S. Department of Health and Human Services, Office of the Surgeon General. Retrieved from: http://www.surgeongeneral.gov/library/obesityvision/obesityvision2010.pdf

[165] Barlow, S.E. (2007). Expert Committee. Expert committee recommendations regarding the prevention, assessment, and treatment of child and adolescent overweight and obesity: summary report. *Pediatrics, 120* (Supplemental 4), S1 64-92.

[166] Brownell, K. and Puhl, R. (2003). Stigma and Discrimination in Weight Management and Obesity. *The Permanente Journal 7*(3), 21-23.

[167] Puhl, R.M., Latner, J.D. (2007). Stigma, obesity, and the health of the nation's children. *Psychological Bulletin 133*(4), 557-80.

[168] Barlow, S.E. (2007). Expert Committee. Expert committee recommendations regarding the prevention, assessment, and treatment of child and adolescent overweight and obesity: summary report. *Pediatrics, 120* (Supplemental 4), S164-92.

[169] Barlow, S.E. (2007). Expert Committee. Expert committee recommendations regarding the prevention, assessment, and treatment of child and adolescent overweight and obesity: summary report. *Pediatrics, 120* (Supplemental 4), S1 64-92.

[170] U.S. Preventive Services Task Force. (2010). Screening for Obesity in Children and Adolescents: U.S. Preventive Services Task Force Recommendation Statement. *Pediatrics, 125*, 361-367. Retrieved from: http://www.ahrq.gov/CLINIC/uspstf/uspschobes.htm.

[171] Section 4004 ("Education and Outreach Campaign Regarding Preventive Benefits") of the Patient Protection and Affordable Care Act of 2010, Pub. L. no 111-148.

[172] Section 1001 ("Sec. 2713. Coverage of Preventive Health Services") of the Patient Protection and Affordable Care Act of 2010, Pub. L. no 111-148.

[173] U.S. Department of Education, National Center for Education Statistics. (2009). *Projections of Education Statistics to 2018, Table 1: Actual and projected numbers for enrollment in grades PK–12, PK–8, and 9–12 in elementary and secondary schools, by control of school: Fall 1993 through fall 2018.* Washington, D.C.: U.S. Government Printing Office. Retrieved from http://nces.ed.gov/programs/projections/projections2018/index.asp.

[174] Silva, E. (2007). *On the Clock: Rethinking the Way Schools Use Time.* Washington, DC: Education Sector, 2007.

[175] U.S. Department of Agriculure. Program Administrative Data. Unpublished.

[176] Gordon, A. et al. (2007). *Dietary Assessment Study-III.* Alexandria, VA: U.S. Department of Agriculture, Food and Nutrition Service, Office of Research, Nutrition and Analysis, School Nutrition.

[177] Gordon, A. et al. (2007). *Dietary Assessment Study-III.* Alexandria, VA: U.S. Department of Agriculture, Food and Nutrition Service, Office of Research, Nutrition and Analysis, School Nutrition.

[178] Institute of Medicine. (2010). *School Meals: Building Blocks for Healthy Children.* Washington, D.C.: The National Academies Press.

[179] Mancino, L., Guthrie, J. (2009). Nudging in the Lunch Line. *Amber Waves, 7*(1). Retrieved from: http://www.ers.usda.gov/AmberWaves/March09/Features/LunchLine.htm.

[180] School Nutrition Association. (2010, February, 9). *SNA Partners with First Lady Michelle Obama's Childhood Obesity Initiative.* [Press Release]. Retrieved from: http://schoolnutrition.org/Blog.aspx?id=13585&blogid=564

[181] Kubik, M. et al. (2003). The association of the school food environment with dietary behaviors of young adolescents. *American Journal of Public Health, 93*(7), 1168–1173; Templeton, S. et al. (2005). Competitive foods increase the intake of energy and decrease the intake of certain nutrients by adolescents consuming school lunch. *Journal of the American Dietetic Association, 105*(2), 21 5–220.

[182] Institute of Medicine. (2007). *Nutrition Standards for Foods in Schools: Leading the Way toward Healthier Youth.* Washington, D.C.: The National Academies Press, 85.

[183] Government Accountability Office. (2005). *School Meal Programs: Competitive Foods are Widely Available and Generate Substantial Revenue for Schools.* GAO-05-563. Washington, D.C.: Government Printing Office, 26-33.

[184] U.S. Department of Agriculture, Food and Nutrition Service, U.S. Department of Health and Human Services, Centers for Disease Control and Prevention, and U.S. Department of Education. (2005). *Making It Happen! School Nutrition Success Stories.* FNS-374. Alexandria, V.A.: U.S. Department of Agriculture.

[185] Kubik, M. et al. (2003). The association of the school food environment with dietary behaviors of young adolescents. *American Journal of Public Health, 93*(7), 1168-1173.

[186] Cullen, K.W., et al. (2008) Improvements in Middle School Student Dietary Intake after Implementation of the Texas Public School Nutrition Policy. *American Journal of Public Health, 98*, 111-117.

[187] Grocery Manufacturers Association. (2010). GMA Statement on Standards for School Foods. [Press Release]. Retrieved from: http://www.gmaonline.org/news/docs/NewsRelease.cfm?DocID=1988&.; American Beverage Association. (2010). Beverage Industry Applauds Members of Congress for Their Leadership on School Nutrition. [Press Release]. Retrieved from: http://www.ameribev.org/news--media

[188] Institute of Medicine. (2007). *Nutrition Standards for Foods in Schools: Leading the Way toward Healthier Youth.* Washington, D.C.: The National Academies Press, 85.

[189] Lee, S.M., Burgeson, C.R., Fulton, J.E., Spain, C.G. (2007). Physical education and physical activity: results from the School Health Policies and Programs Study 2006. *Journal of School Health, 77*, 435-63.

[190] For example, Luepker, R.V., et al. (1996). Outcomes of a field trial to improve children's dietary patterns and physical activity. The Child and Adolescent Trial for Cardiovascular Health. CATCH Collaborative Group. *Journal of the American Medical Association, 275*(1 0), 768–776; Shaya, F.T., Flores, D., Gbarayor, C.M., Wang, J. (2008). School-based obesity interventions: A literature review. *Journal of School Health, 78*(4), 189-196; Contento, I.R., Koch, P.A., Lee, H., Sauberli, W., Calabrese-Barton, A. (2007). Enhancing personal agency and competence in eating and moving: formative evaluation of a middle school

curriculum—Choice, Control, and Change. *Journal of Nutrition Education and Behavior, 39*(5 Supplemental), S179-186.

[191] Just, D.R., Wansink, B., Mancino, L., Guthrie, J. (2008). Behavioral Economic Concepts To Encourage Healthy Eating in School Cafeterias: Experiments and Lessons From College Students, ERR-68. Washington, D.C.: U.S. Department of Agriculture, Economic Research Services; Buergal, N. et al. (2002). Students consuming sack lunches devote more time to eating than those consuming school lunches. *Journal of the American Dietetic Association, 102*(9), 1285.

[192] Wechsler, et al. (1998). Promoting the Selection of Low-Fat Milk in Elementary School Cafeterias in an Inner-City Latino Community: Evaluation of an Intervention. *American Journal of Public Health, 88*, 427-433.

[193] Kavanagh, C. (2009, December). *Flunking Lunch: How Segregated Lunch Lines and Misused Subsidies are Undermining the National School Lunch Program.* Campaign for Better Nutrition. Retrieved from: http://www.campaignforbetternutrition.org/images

[194] Institute Of Medicine. Committee on Food Marketing and the Diets of Children and Youth. (2006). *Food Marketing to Children and Youth, Threat or Opportunity?* Washington, D.C.: The National Academies Press, 187-190; Story, M., French, S. (2004). Food Advertising and Marketing Directed at Children and Adolescents in the US. *International Journal of Behavioral Nutrition and Physical Activity, 1*, 3. Retrieved from: http://www.ijbnpa.org/content/pdf/1479-5868-1-3.pdf.

[195] U.S. Department of Education, National Center for Education Statistics. (2006). *2005–06 School Survey on Crime and Safety, Table 25: Percentage of public high schools reporting use of specified school practices: School year 2005–06.* Washington, D.C.; Government Printing Office, U.S. Department of Education.

[196] Austin, S.B., et al. (2005). Clustering of Fast-Food Restaurants around Schools: A Novel Application of Spatial Statistics to the Study of Food Environments. *American Journal of Public Health, 95*, 1575–1581.

[197] Parmer, S. et al. (2009). School gardens: an experiential learning approach for a nutrition education program to increase fruit and vegetable knowledge, preference, and consumption among second-grade students. *Journal of Nutrition Education and Behavior, 41*(3), 212-7; Ratcliffe, M., Merrigan, K. et al. (2009). The Effects of School Garden Experiences on Middle School-Aged Students' Knowledge, Attitudes, and Behaviors Associated With Vegetable Consumption. Health Promotion Practice.

[198] Kavanagh, C. (2009, December). *Flunking Lunch: How Segregated Lunch Lines and Misused Subsidies are Undermining the National School Lunch Program.* Retrieved from the Campaign for Better Nutrition website, http://www.campaignforbetternutrition.org/images

[199] Story, M., French, S. (2004). Food Advertising and Marketing Directed at Children and Adolescents in the US. *International Journal of Behavioral Nutrition and Physical Activity, 1*, 3. Retrieved from: http://www.ijbnpa.org/content/pdf/1479-5868-1-3.pdf.

[200] Pekruhn, C. (2009). *Preventing Childhood Obesity: A School Health Policy Guide.* Arlington, V.A.: National Association of State Boards of Education, 21.

[201] Parsad, B., Lewis, L. (2009). *Afterschool Programs in Public Elementary Schools.* (NCES 2009-043). Washington, DC: U.S. Department of Education, National Center for Education Statistics, Institute of Education Sciences., 1.

[202] Puzzanchera, C., Adams, B., Sickmund, M. (2010). *Juvenile Court Statistics 2006-2007.* Pittsburgh, PA: National Center for Juvenile Justice.

[203] Sickmund, M. (2010, February). *Juveniles in Residential Placement, 1997-2008.* [Fact Sheet]. Retrieved from the Office of Juvenile Justice and Delinquency Prevention website http://www.ncjrs.gov/pdffiles1/ojjdp/229379.pdf;Hockenberry, S., Sickmund, M., Slad ky, A. (December 2009). *Juvenile Residential Facility Census, 2006: Selected Findings, Juvenile Offenders and Victims: National Report Series.* Washington, D.C.; U.S. Department of Justice Office of Juvenile Justice and Delinquency Prevention, 2.

[204] Gallagher, CA .(2009). Health Care for Juvenile Justice Population. *Georgetown Journal on Poverty Law and Policy, 16*(3) 611; Gallagher, C.A., Dobrin, A. (2007). Can Juvenile Justice Detention Facilities Meet the Call of the American Academy of Pediatrics and National Commission on Correctional Health Care? A National Analysis of Current Practices. *PEDIATRICS, 119*(4); American Academy of Pediatrics .(2001). Health Care for Children and Adolescents in the Juvenile Correctional System, *Pediatrics 107*, 799-800.

[205] Crosby, R. et al. (2003). Health Issues of Juvenile Offenders,In J Moore (Ed.), *Management and administration of correctional health care*(pp. 11-5, 11-8). Kingston, NJ: Civic Research Institute.

[206] Ver Ploeg, M., Breneman, V., Farrigan, T., Hamrick, K., Hopkins, D., Kaufman, P., Lin, B., Nord, M., Smith, T., Williams, R., Kinnison, K., Olander, C., Singh, A., Tuckermanty, E. (2009). *Access to Affordable and Nutritious Food—Measuring and Understanding Food Deserts and Their Consequences: Report to Congress AP-036.* Low- income area is defined as at least 40% of the population with an income below 200% of the federal poverty line.Washington, D.C.: Economic Research Service, U.S. Department of Agriculture.

207 Mikkelsen, L., Chehimi S. (2007). *The Links between the Neighborhood Food Environment and Childhood Nutrition.* Princeton, NJ: Robert Wood Johnson Foundation.

208 Larson, N., Story, M., Nelson M.C. (2009). Neighborhood Environments: Disparities in Access to Healthy Foods in the U.S. *American Journal of Preventive Medicine, 36*(1), 74–81.

209 Van Duyn, M.S., Pivonka, E. (2000). Overview of the Health Benefits of Fruit and Vegetable Consumption for Dietetics Professional: Selected Literature. *Journal of the American Dietetic Association, 100*(12), 1511-1 521.

210 Neumark-Sztainer, D., Story, M., Resnick, M., Blum, R.W. (1996). Correlates of Inadequate Fruit and Vegetable Consumption among Adolescents. *Preventative Medicine, 25*(5), 497-505; Kanh, H.S., Tatham, L.M., Rodriguez, C., Calle, E.E., Thun, M.J., Heatl h, C.W. (1997). Stable Behaviors Associated With Adults' 10-Year Change in Body Mass Index Likelihood of Gain at the Waist. *American Journal of Public Health, 87*(5), 747- 754; Müller, M.J., I Koertzinger, M Mast, K Langnäse, and A Grund (1999). Physical Activity and Diet in 5 to 7 Years Old Children, *Public Health Nutrition, 2*, 443-444; Epstein LH, CC Gordy, HA Raynor, M Beddome, CK Kilanowski, and R Paluch. (2001). Increasing Fruit and Vegetable Intake and Decreasing Fat and Sugar Intake in Families at Risk for Childhood Obesity. *Obesity Research, 9*(3),1 71-178; McCrory MA, Fuss PJ, Saltzman E, and Roberts SB. (2000). Dietary Determinants of Energy Intake and Weight Regulation in Healthy Adults. *Journal of Nutrition, 130*, 276S-279S.

211 Dong, D., Lin, B.H. (2009). *Fruit and Vegetable Consumption by Low-Income Americans: Would a Price Reduction Make a Difference?* ERR-70. Washington, D.C.: U.S. Department of Agriculture.

212 Treuhaft, S., Karpyn, A. (2010). *The Grocery Gap: Who Has Access to Healthy Food and Why It Matters.* Oakland .C.A.: Policy Link and The Food Trust.

213 Powell, L., C Auld, F., Chaloupka, J., O'Malley P.M., Johnston, L.D. (2007). Associations between Access to Food Stores and Adolescent Body Mass Index. *American Journal of Preventive Medicine, 33*(4)Supplement 1, S301-S307.

214 Michigan Department of Community Health's Cardiovascular Health, Nutrition and Physical Activity Section. (n.d.). *Online Home of the Nutrition Environment Assessment Tool (NEAT).* Retrieved from: http://www.mihealthtools.org/neat/

215 Department of Defense, U.S. Navy: Navy & Marine Corps Public Health Center (2009). *Choose Healthy Options for Wellness (CHOW) aka Develop Improved Nutririon Environment (DINE).* Retrieved from: http://www-nehc.med.navy.mil/healthy_living/nutrition

216 Policy Guide on Community and Regional Food Planning. (2007). Retrieved from the American Planning Institute website https://myapa.planning.org/policyguides/food

217 Variyam, J.N. (2005). The Price is Right: Economics and the Rise in Obesity. *Amber Waves 3*(1), 20-27.

218 Based on the seasonally adjusted Consumer Price Index (CPI) for all Urban Consumers in January 1978 and December 2009. The CPI for fruits and vegetables increased from 66.1 to 269.4 over this period; the CPI for carbonated drinks increased from 67.6 to 153.6.

219 Drenowski, A, Specter, S.E. (2004). Drewnowski and Obesity: The Role of Energy Density and Energy Costs. *American Journal of Clinical Nutrition, 79*(1), 6-16; Drenowski, A., Darmon, N. (2005). The Economics of Obesity: Dietary Energy Density and Energy Cost. American Journal of Clinical Nutrition, 82(supplement), 265S-273S.

220 Kuchler, F. et al. (2004). Taxing Snack Foods: What to Expect for Diet and Tax Revenues. *Current Issues in Economic of Food Markets, Agriculture Information Bulletin, 747-08.* Washington D.C.: U.S. Department of Agriculture, Econmic Research Services.

221 Drenowski A., Specter S.E. (2004). Poverty and Obesity: The Role of Energy Density and Energy Costs. *American Journal of Clinical Nutrition, 79*(1), 6-16; Drenowski, A., Darmon N. (2005). The Economics of Obesity: Dietary Energy Density and Energy Cost. American Journal of Clinical Nutrition, 82(supplement), 265S-273S; French S.A. (2003 March). Pricing effects on food choices. Nutrition, 133(3), 841 S-843S.

222 Buzby, J.C., Hodan F.W., Vocke, G. (2006). Possible Implications for U.S. Agriculture from Adoption of Select Dietary Guidelines. *USDA Economic Research Service Report 31*, iii. Retrieved from: http://www.ers.usda.gov/publications/err31/err31.pdf.

223 Miller, J.C., Coble, K.H. (2007). Cheap Food Policy: Fact or Rhetoric? *Food Policy, 32,* 98-111.

224 Based on USDA Economic Research Service comparison of prices paid by consumers for food with prices received by farmers. Price Spreads from Farm to Consumer. (n.d.). Retrieved from: http://www.ers.usda.gov/Data/FarmToConsumer. For processed products the farm value share is even smaller. For example, Economic Research Service data show that the farm value share of corn syrup is only 3.

225 Alston, J.M., Sumner, D.A., Vosti, S.A. (2008). Farm Subsidies and Obesity in the United States: National Evidence and International Comparisons. *Food Policy, 33,* 470–479.

226 Institute of Medicine, Committee on Childhood Obesity Prevention Actions for Local Governments. (2009). *Local Government Actions to Prevent Childhood Obesity.* Washington DC: The National Academy Press; Brownell, K., Frieden, T.R. (2009). Ounces of Prevention — The Public Policy Case for Taxes on Sugared Beverages. *New England Journal of Medicine, 360*(1 8),1 805-1808; Powell, L., Chaloupka, F.J.

(2009). Food Prices and Obesity: Evidence and Policy Implications for Taxes and Subsidies. *The Milbank Quarterly, 87*(1), 229-257.

[227] Andreyeva, T., Long, M., Brownell, K. (2009). The Impact of Food Prices on Consumption: A Systematic Review of Research on Price Elasticity of Demand for Food. *American Journal of Public Health, 100*(2), 216-222.

[228] Powel, L.M., Chriqui, J., Chaloupka, F.J. (2009). Associations between State-level Soda Taxes and Adolescent Body Mass Index. *Journal of Adolescent Health, 45*(3), S57-S63

[229] Fletcher, J.M., Frisvold, D.,Tefft N. (2009). Can Soft Drink Taxes Reduce Population Weight? *Contemporary Economic Policy, 28*(1), 23-35.

[230] Brownell, K., Frieden, T.R. (2009). Ounces of Prevention — The Public Policy Case for Taxes on Sugared Beverages. *New England Journal of Medicine, 360*(1 8),1 805-08; Engelhard, C., Garson, A., Dorn, S. (2009). *Reducing Obesity: Policy Strategies from the Tobacco Wars.* Washington, DC: The Urban Institute.

[231] French, S.A. (2003). Pricing Effects on Food Choices. *Journal of Nutrition, 133*, 841 S-843S;French, S.A., Jeffery, R., Story, M., Hannan, P., Snyder, M.P. (1997). A Pricing Strategy to Promote Low-Fat Snack Choices through Vending Machines. *American Journal of Public Health, 87*, 849-851; French, S.A., Jeffery, R., Story, M., Breitlow, K.K., Baxter, J.S., Hannan, P., Snyder M.P. (2001). Pricing and Promotion Effects on Low-Fat Vending Snack Purchases: The CHIPS Study. American Journal of Public Health, 91, 112–17.

[232] Garson, A., Engelhard., C.L. (2007). Attacking Obesity: Lessons from Smoking. *Journal of the American College of Cardiology, 49*(16), 1673-75.

[233] Dong, D., Lin, B.H. (2009). *Fruit and Vegetable Consumption by Low-Income Americans: Would a Price Reduction Make a Difference?* ERR-70. Washington, D.C.: U.S. Department of Agriculture, Economic Research Service.

[234] Schumacher, A., Winch, R. Park, A.(2009). *Fresh, Local, Affordable: Nutrition Incentives at Farmers' Markets 2009 Update.* Westport, CT: Wholesome Wave Foundation.

[235] Economic Research Service (ERS), U.S. Department of Agriculture (USDA). (2008). Food Availability (Per Capita) Data System. *Fruit and Vegetable spreadsheet.* Retrieved from: http://www.ers.usda.gov/Data/FoodConsumption/FoodAvailSpreadsheets.htm#fruitveg.

[236] Buzby, J.C., Wells, H.F., Vocke, G. (2006). Possible Implications for U.S. Agriculture From Adoption of Select Dietary Guidelines, ERR-31. U.S. Department of Agriculture, Economic Research Service. Retrieved from: http://www.ers.usda.gov/publications/err31/err31.pdf.

[237] Economic Research Service (ERS), U.S. Department of Agriculture (USDA) (2009). Briefing Room - *Food Marketing System in the U.S.: New Product Introductions.* Retrieved from: http://www.ers.usda.gov/Briefing/FoodMarketingSystem/new_product.htm

[238] Golan, E., Mancino, L., Unnevehr, L. (2009). Check the List of Ingredients. *Amber Waves, 7*(2), 19.

[239] Nord, M., Andrews, M., Carlson, S. (2009). *Household Food Security in the United States, 2008.* ERR-83. Wahsington, D.C.: U.S. Department of Agriculture, Economic Research Service.

[240] Dinour, L.M., Bergen, D., Yeh, M. (2007). The Food Insecurity–Obesity Paradox: A Review of the Literature and the Role Food Stamps May Play. *Journal of the American Dietetic Association, 107*(11), 1952-1961.

[241] Rank, M.R., Hirsch l, T.A. (2009). Estimating the Risk of Food Stamp Use and Impoverishment during Childhood. *Archives of Pediatric and Adolescent Medicine, 163*(11), 994-999.

[242] Cole, N., Fox, M.K. (2008). *Diet Quality of Americans by Food Stamp Participation Status: Data from the National Health and Nutrition Examination Survey* FSP-08-NH. Cambridge, M.A.: Abt Associates, Inc.

[243] Leftin, J., Wol kwitz, K. (2009). *Trends in Supplemental Nutrition Assistance Program Participation Rates: 2000 to 2007.* Retrieved from: http://www.fns.usda.gov/ora/menu/Published/snap/FILES/Participation/Trends2000-2007Sum.pdf

[244] Leftin, J., Wol kwitz, K. (2009). *WIC Eligibles and Coverage – 1994 Trends in Supplemental Nutrition Assistance Program Participation Rates: 2000 to 2007: Estimates of the Population of Women, Infants, and Children Eligible.* Alexandria, VA: U.S. Department of Agriculture, Food and Nutrition Service, Office of Research and Analysis.

[245] U.S. Department of Health and Human Services, Office of Disease Prevention and Health Promotion. (2008). *2008 Physical Activity Guidelines for Americans.* Retrieved from: http://www.health

[246] Department of Health and Human Services, Centers for Disease Control and Prevention, Division of Adolescent and School Health. (n.d.) *Healthy Youth!* Retrieved from: http://www.cdc.gov/healthyyouth/physicalactivity.

[247] Tremblay, M., Inman, J., Williams, J. (2000). The relationship between physical activity, self-esteem, and academic achievement in 12-year-old children. *Pediatric Exercise Science, 12,* 312-323; Calfas, K., Taylor, W. (1994). Effects of physical activity on psychosocial variables in adolescents. Pediatric Exercise Science, 6(4), 406-423.

[248] Shephard, R.J. (1997) Curricular physical activity and academic performance. Pediatric Exercise Science, 9, 113-126; Grissom, J. (2005). Physical fitness and academic achievement. *Journal of Exercise Physiology-online, 8*(1), 11-25; Centers for Disease Control and Prevention. (2010). *The association between school-*

based physical activity, including physical education, and academic performance. Atlanta, GA: U.S. Department of Health and Human Services.

[249] U.S. Department of Health and Human Services, Office of Disease Prevention and Health Promotion. (2008). *2008 Physical Activity Guidelines for Americans.* Retrieved from: http://www.health

[250] Outdoor Industry Foundation. (2004). Exploring the active lifestyle: Executive Summary. Retrieved from: http://www.outdoorfoundation.org/pdf/ResearchActiveLifestyleExecutive.pdf

[251] U.S. Department of Health and Human Services, Office of Disease Prevention and Health Promotion. (2008). *2008 Physical Activity Guidelines for Americans.* Retrieved from: http://www.health

[252] Trost, S.G., Pate, R.R., Ward, D.S., Saunders, R., Riner, W. (1999). Correlates of objectively measured physical activity in preadolescent youth. *American Journal of Preventive Medicine, 17,* 120-6.

[253] Sallis, J.F., Prochaska, J.J., Taylor, W.C. (2000). A review of correlates of physical activity of children and adolescents. *Medicine and Science in Sports and Exercise, 32,* 963-75; Van der Horst, K., Paw, M.J., Twisk, J.W., Van Mechelen, W. (2007). A brief review on correlates of physical activity and sedentariness in youth. *Medicine and Science in Sports and Exercise, 39,* 1241-50; Dowda, M., Dishman, R., Pfeiffer, K.A., Pate, R. (2006). Family support for physical activity in girls from 8th to 12th grade in South Carolina. *Preventative Medicine, 44,* 153-9; Heitzler, C.D., Martin, S.L., Duke, J., Huhman, M. (2006). Correlates of physical activity in a national sample of children aged 9-13 years. *Preventative Medicine, 42,* 254-60; Trost, S., Sallis, J., Pate, R., Freedson, P., Taylor, W., Dowda, M. (2003). Evaluating a model of parental influence on youth physical activity. *American Journal of Preventive Medicine, 25,* 277-82.

[254] Centers for Disease Control and Prevention. (2007). *National Youth Risk Behavior Surveillance—United States, 2007.* Unpublished data.

[255] Kaiser Family Foundation. (2010). Generation M2: Media in the Lives of 8- to 18-Year-Olds. Retrieved from: http;//www.kff.org/entmedia/upload/801 0.pdf.

[256] Centers for Disease Control and Prevention. *National Youth Risk Behavior Surveillance—United States, 2007.* Unpublished data.

[257] Steele CA, Kalins IV, Rossen BE, Biggar DW, Bortolussi JA, Jutai JW. (2004). Age-related health risk behaviors of adolescents with physical disabilities. *Soz-Praventivmed 49,* 132–141.

[258] Rimmer, J.H., Rowland, J.A. (2008). Physical activity for youth with disabilities: A critical need in an underserved population. *Developmental Neurorehabilitation, 11*(2), 141–148.

[259] Rimmer, J.H., Rowland, J.A. (2008). Physical activity for youth with disabilities: A critical need in an underserved population. *Developmental Neurorehabilitation, 11*(2), 141–148.

[260] Livsey, S., Hockenberry, S., Knoll, C,, Sladky, A., Sickmund, M. (2010). Required and Voluntary Exercise: *A Special Analysis of Juvenile Residential Facility Census 2008 Data.* Pittsburgh, PA: National Center for Juvenile Justice.

[261] Institute of Medicine. (2005). *Preventing Childhood Obesity: Health in the Balance.* Washington, DC: The National Academies Press; Sallis J., Glanz, K. (2009). Physical Activity and food environments: Solutions to the obesity epidemic. *The Millbank Quarterly 87*(1), 123-54.

[262] Institute of Medicine, Committee on Childhood Obesity Prevention Actions for Local Governments. (2009). *Local Government Actions to Prevent Childhood Obesity.* Washington DC.: The National Academies Press.

[263] Stanford School of Medicine. (2007). Building "Generation Play": *Addressing the Crisis of Inactivity Among America's Children.* Stanford, C.A.: Stanford University..

[264] National Association for Sport and Physical Education. (2005). *Understanding the difference: is it physical education or physical activity?* Reston, V.A.: National Association for Sport and Physical Education, 1-2; National Association for Sport and Physical Education. (2008). *Comprehensive school physical activity programs.* Reston, VA, National Association for Sport and Physical Education, 1-11.

[265] National Association for Sport and Physical Education. (2004). *Moving into the future: national standards for physical education* (2 ed). Reston, V.A.: National Association for Sport and Physical Education; National Association for Sport and Physical Education. (2001). *Physical education is critical to a complete education.* Reston, V.A.: National Association for Sport and Physical Education.

[266] Centers for Disease Control and Prevention. (2010). *The association between school-based physical activity, including physical education, and academic performance.* Atlanta, GA: U.S. Department of Health and Human Services.

[267] Michigan State Board of Education. (2005). Model Local Wellness Policy. Retrieved from: http://www.michigan.gov/documents/Policy_on_Welness_141434_7.pdf.

[268] Chriqui JF, Schneider L, Chaloupka FJ, Ide K and Pugach O. (2009). *Local Wellness Policies: Assessing School District Strategies for Improving Children's Health, School Years 2006-07 and 2007-08.* Chicago, IL: Bridging the Gap Program, Health Policy Center, Institute for Health Research and Policy, University of Illinois at Chicago.

[269] Belansky, E., Cutforth, N., Delong, E., Ross, C., Scarbro, S., Gilbert, L., Beatty, B., Marshall, J. (2009). Early impact of the Federally mandated Local Wellness Policy on physical activity in rural, low-income elementary schools in Colorado. *Journal of Public Health Policy, 30,* S141–S160.

[270] Luepker, R.V., Perry, C.L., McKinlay, S.M., Nader, P.R., Parcel, G.S., Stone, E.J. et al. (1996). Outcomes of a field trial to improve children's dietary patterns and physical activity. The Child and Adolescent Trial for Cardiovascular Health. *Journal of the American Medical Association, 275*, 768-76; Trudeau, F., Shephard, R.J. (2005). Contribution of school programmes to physical activity levels and attitudes in children and adults. *Sports Medicine, 35*, 89-105; McKenzie, T.L., Nader, P.R., Strikmiller, P.K., Yang, M., Stone, E.J., Perry, C.L. et al. (1996). School physical education: effect of the Child and Adolescent Trial for Cardiovascular Health. *Preventative Medicine, 25*, 423-31; McKenzie, T.L., Marshall, S.J., Sallis, J.F., Conway, T.L. (2000). Student activity levels, lesson context, and teacher behavior during middle school physical education. *Research Quarterly for Exercise & Sport, 71*, 249-59; Sal lis, J.F., McKenzie, T.L., Alcaraz, J.E., Kolody, B., Faucette, N., Hovel l, M.F. (1997). The effects of a 2-year physical education program (SPARK) on physical activity and fitness in elementary school students. Sports, Play, and Active Recreation for Kids. *American Journal of Public Health, 87*, 1328-34.

[271] Trudeau, F., Shephard, R.J. (2005). Contribution of school programmes. *Sports Medicine, 35*, 89-105; Dishman, R.K., Motl, R.W., Saunders, R., Felton, G., Ward, D.S., Dowda, M. et al. (2005). Enjoyment mediates effects of a school-based physical-activity intervention. *Medicine and Science in Sports and Exercise, 37*, 478- 87.

[272] Gordon-Larsen, P., McMurray, R.G., Popkin, B.M. (2000). Determinants of adolescent physical activity and inactivity patterns. *Pediatrics, 105*, E83-E91.

[273] Kahn, E.B., Ramsey, L.T., Brownson, R.C., Heath, G.W., Howze, E.H., Powell, K.E. et al. (2002). The effectiveness of interventions to increase physical activity. A systematic review. *American Journal of Preventive Medicine , 22*(Supplement 4), 73-1 07.

[274] National Association for Sport and Physical Education. (2001). *Physical education is critical to a complete education.* Reston, V.A.: National Association for Sport and Physical Education; National Association for Sport and Physical Education. (2004). *Moving into the future: national standards for physical education* (2 ed). Reston, V.A.: National Association for Sport and Physical Education.

[275] National Association for Sport and Physical Education. (2004). *Moving into the future: national standards for physical education* (2 ed). Reston, V.A.: National Association for Sport and Physical Education; Kahn, E.B., Ramsey, L.T,, Brownson, R.C., et al. (2002). The effectiveness of interventions to increase physical activity: a systematic review. American Journal of Preventative Medicine, 22(Supplement 4), 73-107.

[276] Lee SM, Burgeson CR, Fulton JE, Spain CG. Physical education and physical activity: results from the School Health Policies and Programs Study 2006. J Sch Health 2007;77:435-63

[277] Papacharisis, V., Goudas, M. (2003). Perceptions about exercise and intrinsic motivation of students attending a health-related physical education program. *Perceptual and Motor Skills, 97*, 689-96; Daley, A.J., Buchana, J. (1999). Aerobic dance and physical self-perceptions in female adolescents: some implications for physical education. *Research Quarterly for Exercise & Sport, 70*, 196-200.

[278] Dishman, R.K., Motl, R.W., Saunders, R., Felton, G., Ward, D.S., Dowda, M. et al. (2005). Enjoyment mediates effects of a school-based physical-activity intervention. *Medicine and Science in Sports and Exercise, 37*, 478-87; Dishman RK. (2005). Self-management strategies mediate self-efficacy and physical activity. *American Journal of Preventive Medicine, 29*, 10-18.

[279] Sallis J, Prochaska J, Taylor W. (2005). A review of correlates of physical activity of children and adolescents. *Medicine and Science in Sports and Exercise, 32*(5): 963-975.

[280] Lee, S.M,, Burgeson, C.R.,, Fulton, J.E., Spain, C.G. (2007). Physical education and physical activity: results from the School Health Policies and Programs Study 2006. *Journal of School Health, 77*, 435-63.

[281] Dwyer, T., Sallis, J.F., Blizzard, L., Lazarus, R., Dean, K. (2001). Relation of academic performance to physical activity and fitness in children. *Pediatric Exercise Science, 13*, 225-37.

[282] Centers for Disease Control and Prevention. (2010). *The association between school-based physical activity, including physical education, and academic performance.* Atlanta, GA: U.S. Department of Health and Human Services.

[283] Sepia (2009, August 12). Dropped Ball. *Orlando Sentinel.*

[284] Ridgers, N.D., Stratton, G., Fairclough S.J. (2006). Physical activity levels of children during school playtime. *Sports Medicine, 36*, 259-71; Ridgers, N.D., Stratton, G., Fairclough, S.J. (2005). Assessing physical activity during recess using accelerometry. *Prev Med,41*,102-7; Zask, A., Van Beurden, E., Barnett, L., Brooks, L.O., Dietrich, U.C. (2001). Active school playgrounds--myth or reality?: Results of the "move it groove it" project. *American Journal of Preventative Medicine, 33*, 402-8.

[285] National Association for Sport and Physical Education. (2006). *Recess in Elementary Schools.* Reston: National Association for Sport and Physical Education; Burdette, H.L., Whitaker, R.C. (2005). Resurrecting free play in young children: looking beyond fitness and fatness to attention, affiliation, and affect. *Archives of Pediatric Adolescent Medicine, 159*, 46-50.

[286] Centers for Disease Control and Prevention. (2010). *The association between school based physical activity, including physical education, and academic performance.* Atlanta, GA: U.S. Department of Health and Human Services.

[287] Bergman, E., Buergel, N., Englund, T., Femrite, A. (2004). The relationship between recess and meal schedules to plate waste in elementary schools. *Journal of Child Nutrition and Management, 2.*

[288] Lee, S.M,, Burgeson, C.R.,, Fulton, J.E., Spain, C.G. (2007). Physical education and physical activity: results from the School Health Policies and Programs Study 2006. *Journal of School Health, 77*, 435-63..

[289] U.S. Department of Education, National Center for Education Statistics. (2005). *Calories in, calories out.* Washington, D.C.: Food and Exercise in Public Elementary Schools.

[290] Stewart, J.A., Dennison, D.A., Kohl, H.W., Doyle, J.A. (2004). Exercise level and energy expenditure in the TAKE 10! in-class physical activity program. *Journal of School Health, 74*, 397-400.

[291] Mahar, M.T., Murphy, S.K., Rowe, D.A., Golden, J., Shields, A., Raedeke, T.D. (2006). Effects of a classroom-based program on physical activity and on-task behavior. *Medicine and science in sports and exercise, 238*, 2086-94.

[292] National Institutes of Health, National Heart, Lung, and Blood Institute. *National Asthma Education and Prevention Program.* Retrieved from: http://www.nhlbi.nih.gov/health

[293] Farbman, David. (2009). *Tracking an Emerging Movement: A Report on Expanded- Time Schools in America. Boston: National Center on Time and Learning.* Retrieved from: http://www.timeandlearning.org/databasefullreport2009.html.

[294] Frazier, J. A., Morrison, F. J. (1998). The Influence of Extended-year Schooling on Growth of Achievement and Perceived Competence in Early Elementary School. *Child Development, 69*, 495–497.

[295] Durla k, J. A., & Weissberg, R. P. (2007). *The impact of after-school programs that promote personal and social skills.* Chicago, IL: Collaborative for Academic, Social, and Emotional Learning.

[296] National Association for Sport and Physical Education. (2001). Guidelines for after-school physical activity and intramural sport programs. Retrieved from: http://www.ncpublicschools.org/docs/curriculum

[297] Lee, SM, Burgeson, CR, Fulton, JE and Spain, CG. (2007). Physical Education and Physical Activity: Results From the School Health Policies and Programs Study 2006. *Journal of School Health, 77*, 435-63.

[298] National Association for Sport and Physical Education. (2001). *Guidelines for after-school physical activity and intramural sport programs.* Reston, VA: National Association for Sport and Physical Education.

[299] Gordon-Larsen, P. et al. (2000). Determinants of adolescent physical activity and inactivity patterns. *PEDIATRICS 105*(6), E83-E91. Retrieved from: http://pediatrics.aappublications.org/cgi/content/abstract/105/6/e83; Sal lis, J.F., McKenzie, T.L., Conway, T.L., Elder, J.P., Prochaska, J.J., Brown, M. et al. (2003). Environmental interventions for eating and physical activity: a randomized controlled trial in middle schools. *American Journal Preventative Medicine, 24*, 209-17.

[300] National Policy and Legal Analysis Network to Prevent Childhood Obesity. (2009). What is a joint use agreement? *National Policy and Legal Analysis Network to Prevent Childhood Obesity.* Retrieved from: http://www.nplanonline.org/system/files/nplan/JointUse_FactSht_FINAL_web

[301] Farley, T., Meriwether, R., Baker, E., Watkins, L., Johnson, C., Webber L. (2007). Safe play spaces to promote physical activity in inner-city children: Results from a pilot study of an environmental intervention. *American Journal of Public Health, 97*, 1625–1631.

[302] National Association for Sport and Physical Education. (2004). *Moving into the future: national standards for physical education* (2 ed). Reston, V.A.: National Association for Sport and Physical Education; National Association for Sport and Physical Education. (2001). *Physical education is critical to a complete education.* Reston, V.A.: National Association for Sport and Physical Education.

[303] Harrison, P., Gopalakrishnan, N. (2003). Differences in behavior, psychological factors, and environmental factors associated with participation in school sports and other activities in adolescence. *Journal of School Health, 73*, 113-120; Vil hjalmsson, R., Kristjansdottir, G. (2003). Gender differences in physical activity in older children and adolescents: The central role of organized sport. *Social Science Medicine, 56*, 363-374; Katzmarzyk, P., Malina, R. (2000). Contribution of organized sports participation to estimated daily energy expenditure in youth. *Pediatric Exercise Science, 13*, 378-385.

[304] Boreham, C., Twisk, J., Savage, M., Cran, G., Strain, J. (1997). Physical activity, sports participation, and risk factors in adolescents. *Medicine & Science in Sports & Exercise, 29*, 788-793.

[305] Pate, R., Trost, S., Levin, S., et al. (2000). Sports participation and health-related behaviors among United States youth. *Archives of Pediatric Adolescent Medicine, 154*, 904-11; Seefeldt, V., Ewing, M.E. (1997). Youth Sports in America. The President's Council on Physical Fitness and Sports. Research Digest, 2, 1-12.

[306] Kaestner, R. and Xu, X. (201 0). Title IX: Girls' Sports Participation, and Adult Female Physical Activity and Weight. *Evaluation Review, 54*, 152-78; Stevenson, B. (2010). *Beyond the classroom: Using Title IX to measure the return to high school sports: Working Paper No. 15728.* The National Bureau of Economic Research.

[307] Lee, S.M,, Burgeson, C.R.,, Fulton, J.E., Spain, C.G. (2007). Physical education and physical activity: results from the School Health Policies and Programs Study 2006. *Journal of School Health, 77*, 435-63.

[308] Eaton, .DK., Kann, L., Kinchen, S., Shanklin, S., Ross, J., Hawkins, J. et al. (2007). Youth Risk Behavior Surveillance-- United States. *Morbidity and Mortality Weekly Review, 57*, 1-36.

[309] Lepri, K. (2009). The state of youth sports in the United States. Retrieved from: http://www.up2us.org/images

[310] National Federation of State High School Associations. (2009). *High School Today.*

[311] Suffolk University Law Review. (2006). Pay-to-play: A risky and largely unregulated solution to save high school athletic programs from elimination. Retrieved from: http://www.law.suffolk.edu/highlights/stuorgs/lawreview/documents/Rausch_Note_Final.pdf).

[312] The Boston Channel. (2008). *Student Athletes Forced to Pay to Play: Program Costs Passed on to Students.* WCVB Boston. Retrieved from: http://www.thebostonchannel.com/education

[313] McCann, B.A., Ewing, R., (2003). *Measuring the Health Effects of Sprawl: A National Analysis of Physical Activity, Obesity, and Chronic Disease.* Retrieved from the Smart Growth America website http://www.smartgrowthamerica.org/healthreport.html; Zhao, Z., Kaestner, R. (2009). *Effects Of Urban Sprawl On Obesity: Working Paper 15436.* Retrieved from the National Bureau Of Economic Research website http://www.nber.org/papers/w15436

[314] U.S. Department of Transportation Federal Highway Administration Office of Policy. (2009). *National Household Travel Survey.*

[315] Black, J. and Macinko, J. (2008). Neighborhoods and obesity. Nutrition Reviews, 66(1), 2-20; Booth, K., Pinkston, M., Poston, W. (2005). Obesity and the built environment. *Journal of the American Dietetic Association, 105*(Supplemental 5), S110-S117.

[316] Transportation Research Board. (2009). *Driving and the Built Environment: The Effects of Compact Development on Motorized Travel, Energy Use, and CO2 Emissions.* Washington D.C.: National Academy of Sciences.

[317] Dannenberg, A.L., Bhatia, R., Cole, B.L., Dora, C., Fielding, J.E., Kraft, K., McClymont-Peace, D., Mindell, J., Onyekere, C., Roberts, J.A., Ross, C.L., Rutt, C.D., Scott-Samuel, A., Tilson, H.H. (2006). Growing the Field of Health Impact Assessment in the United States: An Agenda for Research and Practice. *American Journal of Public Health, 96*, 262-270.

[318] Singh, G.K., Siahpush, M., Kogan, M.D. (2010). Neighborhood socioeconomic conditions, built environments, and childhood obesity. *Health Affairs, 29*(3), 503-5 12.

[319] Vest, J., Valadez, A. (2005). Perceptions of neighborhood characteristics and leisure-time physical inactivity—Austin/Travis County, Texas. *Morbidity and Mortality Weekly Report, 54*(37), 926-928.

[320] Loukaitou-Sideris, A. (2006). Is it safe to walk?: Neighborhood safety and security considerations and their effects on walking. *Journal of Planning Literature, 20*(3), 219-32.

[321] Alexander, L.M., Inchley, J., Todd, J., et al. (2005). The broader impact of walking to school among adolescents: Seven day accelerometry based study. *British Medical Journal, 331*(7524), 1061–1062; Cooper, A.R., Andersen, L.B., Wedderkopp, N., et al. (2005). Physical activity levels of children who walk, cycle or are driven to school. *American Journal of Preventive Medicine, 29*(3),1 79–184; Fulton, J.E., Shisler, J.L., Yore, M.M., Caspersen, C.J. (2005). Active Transportation to school: Findings from a national survey. *Research Quarterly for Exercise and Sport, 76*(3), 352–357; Saksvig, B.I., Catellier, D.J., Pfeiffer, K., et al. (2007). Travel by walking before and after school and physical activity among adolescent girls. *Archives of Pediatrics and Adolescent Medicine, 161*(2), 153–1 58.

[322] Watson, M., Dannenberg, A. (2008). Investment in Safe Routes to School Projects: Public health benefits for the larger community. *Preventing Chronic Disease, 5*(3), A90; Boarnet, M., Day, K., Anderson, C., et al. (2005). California's Safe Routes to School Program- impacts on walking, bicycling, and pedestrian safety. *Journal of the American Planning Association, 71*(3), 301 –317; Hume, C., Timperio, A., Salmon, J., et al. (2009). Walking and cycling to school: Predictors of increases among children and adolescents." *American Journal of Preventive Medicine, 36*(3), 195–200.

[323] Staunton, C., Hubsmith, D., Kallins, W. (2003). Promoting safe walking and biking to school: The Marin County success story. *American Journal of Public Health, 93*(9), 1431–1434.

[324] Boarnet, M., Day, K., Anderson, C., et al. (2005). California's Safe Routes to School Program impacts on walking, bicycling, and pedestrian safety. *Journal of the American Planning Association, 71*(3), 301–317.

[325] U.S. Travel Data Show Decline In Walking and Bicycling To School Has Stabilized. (2010) Retrieved from the Safe Routes to Schools Website http://www.saferoutesinfo.org/news_room/2010-04-08_2010_nhts_release.cfm.

[326] U.S. Travel Data Show Decline In Walking and Bicycling To School Has Stabilized. (2010) Retrieved from the Safe Routes to Schools Website http://www.saferoutesinfo.org/news_room/2010-04-08_2010_nhts_release.cfm.

[327] Martin, S., Carlson, S. (2004). Barriers to children walking to and from school. *Mortality and Morbidity Weekly Review, 54*(3 8), 949-952.

[328] Pucher, D., Handy. (2009). Infrastructure programs, and policies to increase bicycling. Preventive Medicine, 7(28); Jacobson, P.L. (2007) Safety in numbers: More walkers and bicyclists, safer walking and bicycling. *Injury Prevention, 9*, 205-209.

[329] Floriani, V., Kennedy, C. (2008). Promotion of physical activity in children. *Current Opinion in Pediatrics. 20*(1), 90-95.

[330] Grow, H., Saelens, B., Kerr, J., Durant, N., Norman, G., Sallis, J. (2008). Where are youth active? Roles of proximity, active transport, and built environment. *Medicine and Science in Sports and Exercise, 40*(12), 2071-79; Kaczynski, A., Henderson, K. (2008). Parks and recreation settings and active living: A review of associations with physical activity function and intensity. Journal of Physical Activity and Health, 5(4), 619- 632; Davidson K., Lawson, C. (2006). Do attributes of the physical environment influence children's level of physical activity. *International Journal of Behavioral Nutrition and Physical Activity 3*(19), 1-17.

[331] Roemmich, J., Epstein, L., Raja, S., Yin, L., Robinson, J., Winiewics, D. (2006). Associations of access to parks and recreation facilities with physical activity of young children. *Preventive Medicine, 43*, 437-441.

[332] Cohen, D., McKenzie, T., Sehgal, A., Williamson, S., Golinelli, D., Luries, N. (2007). Contribution of parks to physical activity. *American Journal of Public Health, 97*, 509-514.

[333] Bell, S., Hamilton, V., Montarzino, A., Rothnie, H., Travlou, P., & Alves, S. (2008). Greenspace and quality of life: a critical literature review. Greenspace Scotland. Retrieved from: http://www.greenspacescotland.org.uk/default.asp?page=465; Bell, S., Tyrvainen, L., Sievanen, T, Probstl, U. and Simpson, M. (2007). Outdoor Recreation and Nature Tourism: A European Perspective. Retrieved from: http://landscaperesearch.livingreviews.org/Articles/lrlr-2007/title.html; Maller, C., Townsend, M., St.Leger, L., Henderson-Wilson, C., Pryor, A., Prosser, L., and Moore, M. (2008). The health benefits of contact with nature in a park context: A review of relevant literature. Retrieved from: http://www.parkweb.vic.gov.au/1process_content.cfm?section=99&page=16; Taylor, Andrea Faber, and Frances E. Kuo. (2006). Is Contact with Nature Important for Healthy Child Development? State of the Evidence. In Spencer, C. & Blades, M. (Eds.), *Children and Their Environments: Learning, Using and Designing Spaces.* Cambridge, UK: Cambridge University Press.

[334] Ogden, C.L., Carroll, M., Curtin, L., Lamb, M., Flegal, K. (2010). Prevalence of High Body Mass Index in US Children and Adolescents 2007-2008. Journal of American Medical Association, 303(3), 242-249.

[335] National Wildlife Federation. (2008). Connecting Today's Kids with Nature: A Policy Action Plan. Reston, VA: National Wildlife Federation.

[336] Burdette, H. L., Robert, C., Whitaker. (2005). Resurrecting Free Play in Young Children: Looking Beyond Fitness and Fatness to Attention, Affiliation and Affect. *Archives of Pediatric Adolescent Medicine, 159*, 46-50

[337] Centers for Disease Control and Prevention Division of Adolescent and School Health. (2007). School Health Policies and Programs Study. *Journal of School Health, 77*(8).

[338] Task Force on Community Preventive Services. (2002). Recommendations to increase physical activity in communities. *American Journal of Preventive Medicine, 22*(48), 67-72.

In: Solving Childhood Obesity
Editors: Sarah J. Maier and Natalie E. Brunner

ISBN: 978-1-61209-964-4

Chapter 2

CHILDHOOD OVERWEIGHT AND OBESITY: DATA BRIEF

Amalia K. Corby-Edwards

SUMMARY

In children and adolescents, obesity is defined as being at or above the 95th percentile of the age- and sex-specific body mass index (BMI); overweight is defined as being between the 85th and 94th percentiles, based on growth charts developed by the Centers for Disease Control and Prevention. The National Health and Nutrition Examination Survey has gathered data showing that, over the past three decades, obesity rates have tripled among children and adolescents. Today, about 32% of U.S. children and adolescents between the ages of 2 and 19 are overweight, and more than half of those children are considered obese.

The prevalence of overweight and obesity in children varies by age, race, ethnicity, geographic location, and socioeconomic status. In 2007-2008, 10% of children ages 2 to 5 were obese, while nearly 20% of children ages 6 to 19 were obese. Overweight and obesity are more prevalent among certain minority groups and low-income children. Additionally, states with the highest child and adolescent obesity rates are concentrated in the Southeastern region of the United States. Studies suggest that, while these demographic factors are related to weight, behavioral factors, including energy intake, physical activity, and sedentary behaviors also play a role.

The Obama Administration and Congress have shown a strong interest in developing policies to reverse this trend. Federal policies to address childhood obesity span many departments, including the Departments of Health and Human Services, Education, and Agriculture, among others. Reducing childhood obesity is also a major initiative of the First Lady and the Secretary of Health and Human Services. In May 2010, the President's Task Force on Childhood Obesity released an action plan with a series of recommendations to reduce childhood obesity prevalence to 5% from the current 17% by 2030.

Congress is seeking to address this issue through legislation that promotes nutrition, healthy weight, and fitness, particularly in communities, schools, and federal nutrition programs. Some proposed legislation supports research and support of best practices in both federal and community programs. Others have proposed increased monitoring of BMI by health care providers. This report is designed to provide an overview of the data being used to inform federal obesity policy. It analyzes obesity among children and adolescents, including a discussion of obesity measurement, trends in obesity rates, and differences that exist across gender, race, ethnicity, socioeconomic status, and geographic location.

INTRODUCTION

In children and adolescents, obesity is defined as being at or above the 95th percentile of the age- and sex-specific body mass index (BMI); overweight is defined as being between the 85th and 94th percentiles. Over the past three decades, obesity rates have more than doubled among adults, and tripled among children and adolescents. About 32% of U.S. children and adolescents between the ages of 2 and 19 are overweight, and more than half of those children are considered obese.[1] As these numbers have risen, obesity as a public health issue has gained the attention of some policy makers. Obesity increases mortality risk and is associated with a number of chronic conditions in children, such as diabetes, asthma, and risk factors for heart disease.[2] Obese children are at a greater risk for obesity and other chronic conditions in adulthood.[3] Some researchers believe that today's children may lead shorter lives than their parents due to the negative effects of obesity.[4] In addition to those risks, obesity rates in children and adolescents have raised concerns about increased burden on the healthcare system and the effects of obesity on military readiness.[5]

The current administration has shown a strong interest in developing policies to address childhood overweight and obesity. In January, 2010, the Surgeon General issued "The Surgeon General's Vision for a Healthy and Fit Nation 2010," outlining her vision to address obesity in the United States.[6] Childhood obesity is also a major initiative of the First Lady and the Department of Health and Human Services. The President's Task Force on Childhood Obesity released an action plan with a series of recommendations to reduce childhood obesity to five percent by 2030.[7]

Congress is seeking to address this issue through increased funding for school lunch programs, updating school meal nutrition standards, encouraging "farm-to-school" activities, and broadened coverage and support for school wellness programs. Other proposals address collection of data on student fitness levels, nutrition behavior, and physical activity, in addition to higher physical education standards and required activity time in schools. Some suggest requirements for local education agencies to integrate fitness into the school environment and to disseminate information on physical activity to families. Others have called for nationwide physical education requirements in schools, which are currently determined at the local level.

Overweight and obesity often begin in childhood and adolescence and continue into adulthood. Adults are generally considered capable of understanding how to maintain a healthy weight, and are considered capable of making personal choices, when possible, to control their weight. However, children may not have the tools or capacity to understand or prevent overweight and obesity, and the government often has a larger role in their well-being, through schools, health care, and programs for low-income families. This report analyzes data on obesity among children and adolescents including a discussion of obesity measurement, trends in obesity rates, and differences in rates that exist across gender, race, ethnicity, socioeconomic status, and geographic location.

MEASUREMENT OF CHILDHOOD OVERWEIGHT AND OBESITY

According to the Centers for Disease Control and Prevention (CDC), obesity and overweight are terms used to describe ranges of weight that are higher than what is generally considered healthy for a given height.[8] While several methods are available to measure or estimate overweight and obesity, this report relies on the use of body mass index (BMI) to present the data on childhood overweight and obesity. While BMI is not an exact measure of body fat, as discussed below, it is regarded as an efficient measure of childhood overweight and obesity for population-based data. BMI is presented as the indicator of overweight and obesity in most federally-sponsored studies and reports of children's health, including the National Health and Nutrition Examination Survey (NHANES), and Healthy People 2010. BMI is also the most commonly used clinical screening measure for both child and adult overweight and obesity, and is recommended by the U.S. Preventive Services Task Force (USPSTF) for screening purposes.[9]

Measurement

One aspect of the discussion surrounding childhood overweight and obesity is the issue of measurement. Body mass index (BMI), a number calculated from a person's weight and height, is commonly used to screen for obesity. BMI is considered a reliable, easy, and inexpensive way to screen individuals over age two for possible weight problems. [10] In addition to its use in research and surveillance, BMI is widely used in clinical settings. BMI is not a direct measure of body fat, but research has shown that BMI correlates with direct measures of body fat.[11] BMI is used as a rapid and inexpensive screening tool; however, not all children with a high BMI are overweight or obese. Some children may be heavier due to extra muscle mass, not extra body fat. The CDC recommends that a child with a high BMI be examined by a health care provider to determine if overweight or obesity is a concern.

BMI percentiles are determined using population-based growth charts developed by CDC that show age- and sex-specific BMI. These charts were created using reference populations from several surveys administered by CDC between 1963 and 1994.[12] Consequently, when using BMI as an indicator of overweight and obesity today, the measure is referring to the BMI index levels of individuals based on their age, sex, weight, and height compared to their respective reference populations' BMI distributions from which the index was developed. In children, obesity is defined as being at or above the 95th percentile of the age- and sex-specific body mass index (BMI) relative to those reference populations; overweight, also known as "at risk for obesity," is defined as being between the 85th and 94th percentiles.[13] In most children and adolescents, a BMI level at or above the 95th percentile indicates elevated body fat and reflects the presence or risk of related chronic disease. The most recent NHANES data, including those above the 97th percentile, are presented in **Appendix B**.

Data Sources

Child health data are available from several sources, but the types of data and resulting analyses vary. This report presents data from several sources, including the National Health and Nutrition Examination Survey (NHANES), the Youth Risk Behavior Surveillance System (YRBSS), the Pediatric Nutrition Surveillance System (PedNSS), and the National Survey of Children's Health (NSCH). All data used in this report are collected by the Department of Health and Human Services (HHS) with the intent to monitor the nation's health. Each data source is described below, followed by a general discussion of the strengths and weaknesses of the different types of data collected by these systems. For a more detailed comparison of the data sources, see **Appendix A**.

NHANES

The National Health and Nutrition Examination Survey (NHANES) is a continuous national survey that uses mobile examination centers to conduct in-person interviews, physical examinations, diagnostic tests, and nutritional assessments on a nationally representative sample of about 5,000 people of all ages annually. BMI is calculated from direct measure of height and weight by survey staff. These data are available from 1976 to the present. Because the sample size is relatively small, state-level data for children and adolescents are not available from NHANES.[14]

YRBSS

The Youth Risk Behavior Surveillance System (YRBSS) is comprised of national, state, and local school-based surveys of students in grades 9 through 12. It is designed to monitor six categories of health-risk behaviors, including physical activity and dietary habits, in this age group. Participation is voluntary, and students are asked to complete the questionnaire during one class period. In 2007, approximately 14,000 students participated in YRBSS. Since 1991, the survey has been administered once every two years, and it is designed to be nationally representative of all U.S. students in grades 9 through 12. BMI is calculated based on the responses to questions about age, gender, height, and weight. The sample size is large enough to present state-level data, and data are often available from states, as well as from CDC.[15]

PedNSS

The Pediatric Nutrition Surveillance System (PedNSS) continuously monitors the nutritional status of low-income children in federally funded programs, including the Special Supplemental Nutrition Program for Women, Infants, and Children (WIC), the Early and Periodic Screening, Diagnosis, and Treatment (EPSDT) program, and the Maternal and Child Health Bureau Title V program. In 2008, 43 states, the District of Columbia, Puerto Rico, the

U.S. Virgin Islands, and six Indian Tribal Organizations contributed data on 8 million children from birth to five years of age. Contributors to PedNSS vary from year to year, which can affect the trends and representativeness of the data, published annually. Data on birthweight, breastfeeding, anemia, short stature, underweight, overweight, and obesity are collected for children who attend public health clinics for routine care, nutrition education, and supplemental food. BMI is calculated from these data for children ages two and older.[16]

NSCH

The National Survey of Children's Health (NSCH) is a national telephone survey administered by the Maternal and Child Health Bureau of the Health Services and Resource Administration (HRSA) that is conducted every four years. This survey collects a broad range of information on children's health and well-being, and includes information on the family environment. NSCH data are collected in English and Spanish in a manner that allows for valid state and national level comparisons. In 2007, 91,000 surveys were completed for children and adolescents from birth to age 17. A limitation of NSCH is that it has only been administered twice (in 2003 and 2007) making it challenging to analyze trends. However, HRSA plans to administer the survey again in 2011. BMI calculations are based on parent report of gender, age, weight, and height for children ages two and up.

Choosing a Data Source

Estimates of obesity from each data source are different, due to the methods used to collect the data, and coverage, or population base, of the survey or surveillance system. Each data source provides a unique view of childhood obesity, and each has its strengths and weaknesses. When interpreting the data, policymakers should face consideration of the following key points: (1) Are the data self-reported, or measured directly? (2) Are the data reliable at the state level, national level, or both? (3) Is there any additional information collected that would provide a social context for the data?

NHANES is considered the most reliable national estimate, due to the use of direct measurement of participants, but it cannot be used for state-level estimates due to its sample size. PedNSS is also based on clinical measurement of height and weight, but it only provides data for children under age five who are in federally funded programs. YRBSS and NSCH are based on self- or parent-report of height and weight, which has been shown to underestimate BMI.[17] However, these two surveys have large sample sizes and can be analyzed at the state level. Additionally, NSCH collects data on a large number of family and household characteristics, which can be used to characterize the household environment of obese and overweight children. YRBSS collects risk behavior information, which allows researchers and public health professionals to identify behaviors in adolescents that may contribute to obesity. In this report, NHANES is used to present national data, NSCH is used to present state-level estimates, and PedNSS is used to present data on low-income children in federally funded programs.

PREVALENCE OF CHILDHOOD OVERWEIGHT AND OBESITY

The increase in childhood overweight and obesity has affected certain subsets of the population more than others. For instance, BMI in school-age children (ages 6 to 19) has risen at a higher rate than BMI among children ages 2 to 5. This section includes information on the increase in childhood overweight and obesity among specific age groups, gender, race, ethnicity, and geography.

Variation by Age Group

Based on analysis of the most recent NHANES data, about 32% of U.S. children between the ages of 2 and 19 are overweight, and more than half of those children are considered obese.[18] **Figure 1** shows obesity trends by age group since the 1 960s. According to NCHS, between 1976- 1980 and 1999-2000, the prevalence of obesity increased; between 1999-2000 and 2007-2008, there was no significant trend in obesity for any age group.[19] Obesity prevalence, as shown in **Figure 1**, differs by age group; 10% of children ages 2 to 5 are obese, while nearly 20% of children ages 6 to 19 (school-age children and adolescents) are obese. This difference in preschool and school aged children has increased over time, as obesity rates overall have increased.

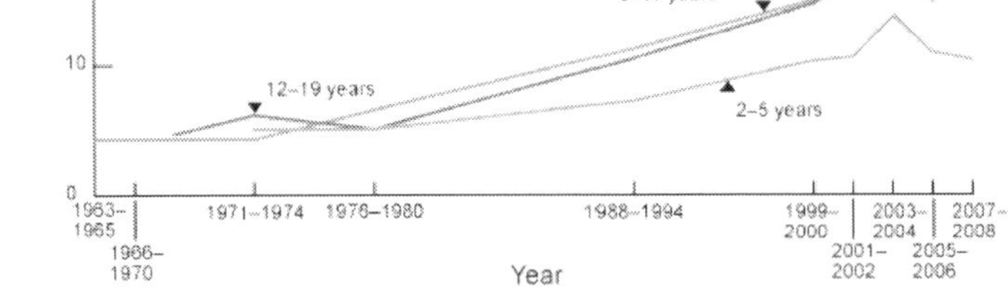

Source: Ogden C, Carroll M, Prevalence of Obesity among Children and Adolescents, United States, Trends 1963-1965 through 2007-2008. NCHS Health E-Stat: http://www.cdc.gov/nchs/data/hestat/obesity obesity_child_07_08.htm.

Notes: CRS did not find any literature to explain the 2003-2004 increase and subsequent decline in 2005-2006. We speculate, however, that it may be attributable to fluctuations in BMI in the study sample, rather than the overall population.

Figure 1. Trends in Obesity among Children and Adolescents, 1963-2008. National Health and Nutrition Examination Survey.

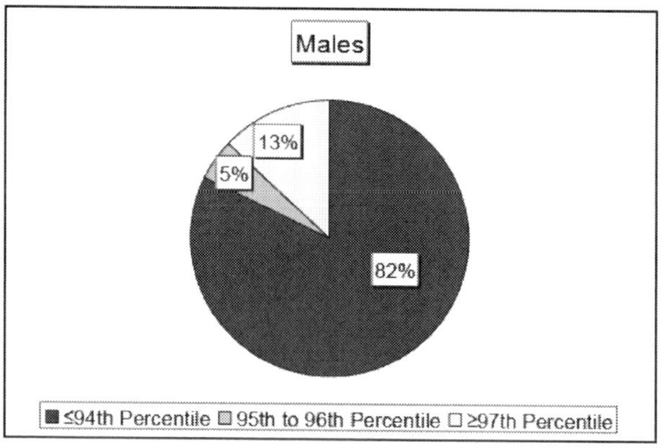

Figure 2. Obesity Prevalence Among Male Children and Adolescents, U.S., 2007-2008.

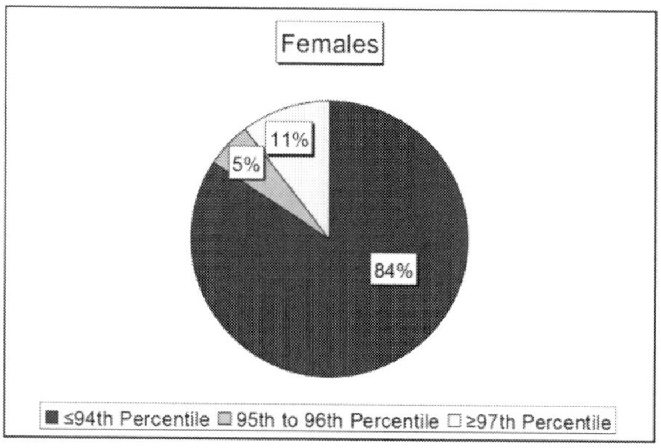

Source: CRS analysis based on data from NHANES as presented in Ogden C, Carroll M, Curtin L, et al., "Prevalence of High Body Mass Index in U.S. Children and Adolescents, 2007-2008," *JAMA*, vol. 303, no. 3 (January 13, 2010), pp. 242-249.

Figure 3. Obesity Prevalence Among Female Children and Adolescents, U.S., 2007-2008.

In *Healthy People 2010*, HHS set a goal of reducing the obesity rate among children and adolescents (ages 6 to 19) to 5% by 2010.[20] While this goal has not been reached, the most recent data show no significant increase in obesity rates overall since 1999.[21] However, except for ages 2 to 5, the rates are not declining, and as seen in **Figure 1**, the rates for ages 6 to 11 have shown an increase in the most recent data. This trend mirrors the trend for adults; after rising steadily in the late 20th century, obesity rates in adults have remained statistically unchanged since 1999.[22]

Variation by Gender, Race, and Ethnicity

Although the rates of obesity have not significantly increased since 1999, there has been a shift among obese children to the higher percentiles. Most children who are obese (95th percentile or above) are at the 97th percentile or above.[23] As shown in **Figure 2** and **Figure 3**, male children are slightly more likely to be obese than females.

Although some variation in BMI is expected between males and females, children and adolescents ages 6 to 19 show the greatest gender gap in obesity rates. Male children and adolescents are also more likely to be at or above the 97th percentile.

The increase in overweight and obese children since 1974 is evident among all age, race, and ethnic groups; however, African American and Hispanic children have been disproportionately affected.[24] Thirty-six percent of non-Hispanic black children and adolescents ages 2 to 19 are overweight or obese, and 38% of Hispanic children and adolescents, compared to 29% of their non-Hispanic white counterparts, as shown in **Appendix C**. **Figure 4** shows that the differences in overweight and obesity by race and ethnicity also vary by age. For example, the proportion of non-Hispanic black adolescents who are overweight or obese is highest for ages 12 to 19, while the proportion of overweight and obese Hispanic and non-Hispanic white children appears to be highest from ages 6 to 11.

Variation by Socioeconomic Status and Geographic Location

Overweight and obesity in children and adolescents has been associated with lower socioeconomic status and geographic location, particularly in the southeastern states.[25] The following section presents some background information on these disparities.

NSCH data indicate that the magnitude of socioeconomic disparities in obesity prevalence may have increased between 2003 and 2007. For example, one analysis indicates that, during this time period, obesity prevalence increased by nearly 25% for children in low-education, low-income, and higher-unemployment households.[26] The same study notes that, in 2007, children from low- income and low-education households had three to four times higher odds of obesity than children from higher socioeconomic households.

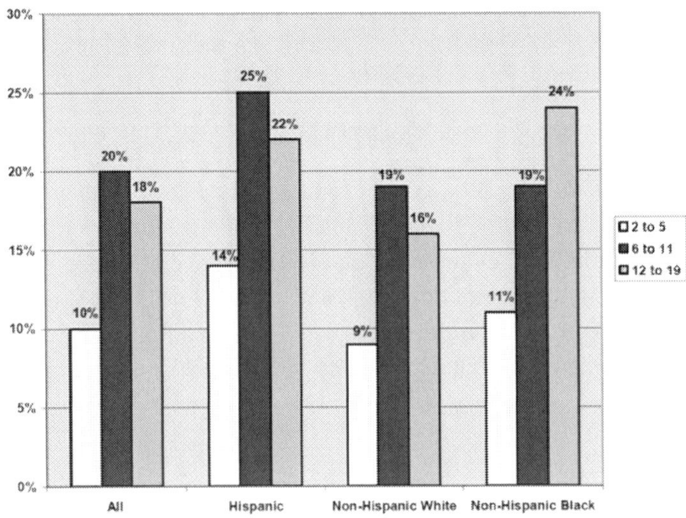

Source: CRS analysis based on data from NHANES (2007-2008) as presented in Ogden C, Carroll M, and Curtin L, et al., "Prevalence of High Body Mass Index in U.S. Children and Adolescents, 2007-2008," *JAMA*, vol. 303, no. 3 (January 13, 2010), pp. 242-249.

Figure 4. Prevalence of Overweight and Obesity in Children and Adolescents by Age and Race/Ethnicity, 2007-2008. National Health and Nutrition Examination Survey, CDC.

Figure 5 presents a map of BMI ranking relative to the nation, by state, of children ages 10 to 17. Parent-reported data on weight and height for younger children are considered less reliable by researchers, and therefore are not presented in the state by state analysis. Prevalence of overweight and obesity was highest in Mississippi (44.5%), and lowest in Utah (23.1%). The five states (Kentucky, Tennessee, Georgia, Arkansas, and Mississippi) with overweight and obesity prevalence that is statistically significantly higher than the U.S. average are all located in the southeastern region.

Obesity among Low-Income Children in Federally Funded Programs

The health status of low-income, preschool-aged children in federally-funded programs is monitored by the CDC's Pediatric Nutrition Surveillance System (PedNSS). Data show that obesity among children in federally-funded programs increased from 12.4% in 1998 to 14.5% in 2003, and remained stable at 14.6% in 2008.[27] The highest prevalence of obesity was found among Hispanic children at 18.5% and American Indian/Alaska Native (AI/AN) children at 21.2%; the lowest prevalence of obesity was among non-Hispanic black children (11.8%) and Asian/Pacific Islander children (12.3%). Non-Hispanic white children had an obesity prevalence of 12.6%. The PedNSS also showed an overall stabilization of obesity rates from 2003 to 2008, with the exception of AI/AN children.

Factors Associated with Childhood Overweight and Obesity

At the individual level, obesity is thought to be caused by a number of interacting genetic, behavioral, and environmental factors.[28] Some behavioral and environmental factors associated with childhood obesity are modifiable at the individual or family level, including energy intake, physical activity, and sedentary activity. Research shows that children who watch more than 2 hours of television per day had a 52% higher risk of obesity than children who watched less than one hour per day. Additionally, children who are not physically active have a 37% higher risk of obesity than those who exercise five days per week.[29] Certain risk factors are also modifiable at the community level, including community and school-based physical activity, and access to healthy foods. One study notes that children ages 10-17 who live in neighborhoods with the most unfavorable social conditions, such as unsafe surroundings, poor housing, and no access to sidewalks, parks, and recreation centers have 20% to 60% higher odds of being obese than children who live in neighborhoods with more favorable social conditions.[30]

Some maternal factors have been associated with childhood obesity; breastfeeding has been associated with lower rates of pediatric obesity.[31] Other factors, such as very low or very high birth weight, maternal smoking, and maternal obesity have been associated with a higher risk of obesity in other studies.

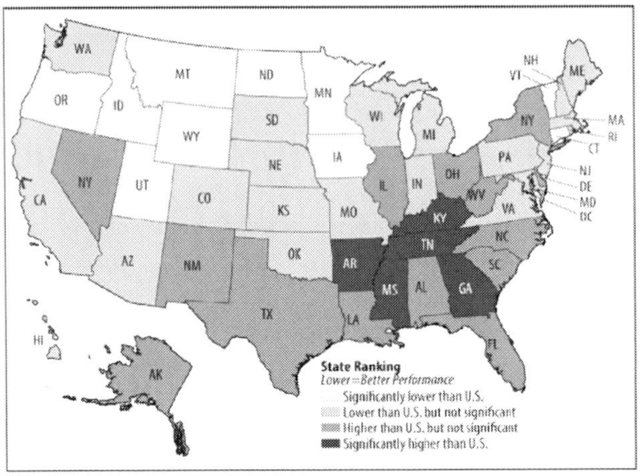

Source: National Survey of Children's Health, 2007 at http://nschdata.org/Rankings/RankingMap.aspx?item= 07 _ind1 _4a.

Notes: Ranking is based on percent of children in each state who are at or above the 85th percentile for BMI.

Figure 5. Obese and Overweight Children and Adolescents Age 1 0 to 17, by State National Survey of Children's Health, Maternal and Child Health Bureau.

RISKS OF CHILDHOOD OVERWEIGHT AND OBESITY

Childhood and adolescent obesity has consequences that may last into adulthood. Youth who are overweight or obese have a higher risk of developing high blood pressure, high cholesterol, and abnormal glucose tolerance, which are risk factors for developing cardiovascular disease later in life.[32] Other health conditions associated with obesity are asthma, hepatic steatosis (i.e., fatty liver), sleep apnea, and Type 2 diabetes.[33] Children with these conditions also have a higher risk of disability.

Increasing rates of childhood chronic conditions may also lead to increases in long-term health burdens among adults, along with increasing medical and disability costs, and decreased work force participation. After age 6, obese children may have a 50% greater chance of becoming obese adults, regardless of their parents' obesity status.[34] Obesity in adults is associated with increased risk of a number of conditions, including diabetes, cardiovascular disease, hypertension, and certain cancers.

The National Institutes of Health has determined that obesity and overweight combined are the second leading cause of preventable death in the United States.[35] In one study, poor diet and physical inactivity were found to be the second-highest actual cause of death, behind tobacco use.[36] Another recent study of American Indians showed that elevated BMI in childhood was associated with a higher risk of premature death.[37] This long-term study of American Indian children found that those in the highest BMI quartile had more than double the risk of premature death than those in the lowest quartile.

Finally, children and adolescents who are overweight may also have social issues; they may be subject to social discrimination, which has long-term effects on self-esteem.[38] Overweight and obese children are less likely to be engaged in school, more likely to repeat a grade in school, and more likely to miss two or more weeks of school per year.[39]

Conclusion

Healthy People 2010 set a number of goals for childhood and adolescent overweight and obesity, including a goal to reduce the proportion of children and adolescents who are overweight or obese to 5%; this goal has not been achieved. While no individual survey or surveillance system can provide the complete picture, the data consistently show that the prevalence of obesity among children and adolescents remains high, particularly among school-age children and among children in federally funded programs.

Childhood obesity is a complex and multi-faceted issue that has been addressed by a wide variety of policies. Policies to address childhood obesity encompass education and health communication, policy development and support at the state and community level, scientific and public health research, and delivery of services including nutrition programs. The data sources discussed in this report are useful decision-making tools for these programs, as well as the Administration and Congress.

Some have called for new policies to address nutrition and physical activity in schools as a major component of addressing childhood obesity. Congress is seeking to address this issue through increased funding for school lunch programs, updating school meal nutrition standards, encouraging "farm-to-school" activities, broadened coverage and support for school wellness programs. These themes are discussed in greater detail in CRS Report R41354, Child Nutrition and WIC Reauthorization: Issues and Legislation in the 111th Congress, by Joe Richardson. Other proposals address collection of data on student fitness levels, nutrition behavior, and physical activity, in addition to higher physical education standards and required activity time in schools. Some suggest requirements for local education agencies to integrate fitness into the school environment and to disseminate information on physical activity to families. Others have called for nationwide physical education requirements in schools, which are currently determined at the local level.

Research has suggested a comprehensive, multi-pronged approach to childhood overweight and obesity. Many projects have been funded and implemented at the community level through federal grants.[40] The Patient Protection and Affordable Care Act (P.L. 111-148) appropriated $25 million for a Childhood Obesity Demonstration Project that was authorized in the 2009 CHIP reauthorization (P.L. 111-3). This demonstration project will provide funding for the development of a comprehensive and systematic model for reducing childhood obesity, through targeted support to families, the identification of behavioral risk factors, identification of needed clinical preventive, screening benefits, and medical assistance.

Congress' actions appear to be generally consistent with the current administration's objectives. HHS is currently finalizing Healthy People 2020 goals. New proposed objectives include reducing the amount of calories children and adolescents get from foods with added fat and sugars; increasing the number of physicians who regularly measure BMI; incentivizing food retail outlets to offer options that follow the dietary guidelines; and increasing state nutrition standards for meals at childcare centers and schools. It is expected that these goals will align with the goals of the President's Task Force on Childhood Obesity.

Appendix A. Data Sources Used in this Report

Table A-1. Characteristics of the NSCH, PedNSS, YRBSS, and NHANES.

	NSCH	PedNSS	YRBSS	NHANES
Description	NSCH is a nationally representative telephone survey on a variety of physical, emotional, and behavioral child health indicators, information on the child's family context and neighborhood environment.	PedNSS is a clinic-based surveillance system that provides data on the prevalence and trends of nutrition-related indicators of low-income U.S. children.	YRBSS is a nationally representative survey designed to monitor priority health-risk behaviors and the prevalence of obesity and asthma among youth and young adults.	NHANES is a nationally representative survey designed to study national health trends and data
Survey Universe	All children and adolescents under 18 years of age	Children age birth to 5 who attend federally funded maternal and child health and nutrition programs.	Students in grades 9-12	All persons
Frequency	Every four years	Continuous	Every two years	Continuous
Survey Years	2003, 2007	Began in 1999	Began in 1990	Began in the 1960s as a series of surveys; in 1999 it became a continuous survey
Annual Sample Size	Approximately 91,000 in 2007	Approximately 8 million children in 2008	Approximately 14,000 students in 2007	Approximately 5,000 persons
Survey Mode	Telephone survey	Existing data from the Special Supplemental Nutrition Program for Women, Infants, and Children (WIC); Early and Periodic Screening, Diagnosis, and Treatment (EPSDT) Program; and Title V Maternal and Child Health Program (MCH).	Self-administered questionnaire	In-person interviews and physical examinations

	NSCH	PedNSS	YRBSS	NHANES
Available Geographies Collected Demographics	Nation and states	Nation and states[c]	Nation and states[c]	Nation only
Age	Children from birth through age 17	Children from birth through age 4	Students in grades 9-12	All ages
Gender	Male and Female	Male and Female	Male and Female	Male and Female
Race	White, Black, Asian, NHOPI,[a] AIAN,[b] Other	White, Black, Asian, NHOPI[a] , AIAN[b], Other	White, Black, Asian, NHOPI,[a] AIAN,[b] Other	White, Black, Asian, NHOPI,[a] AIAN,[b] Other
Ethnicity	Hispanic/Latino	Hispanic/Latino	Hispanic/Latino	Hispanic/Latino
Obesity Data Collection Process	Respondents self- report height and weight and the CDC uses the measurements to calculate each respondents' BMI	Medical personnel measure respondents' height and weight to calculate weight for length or BMI as part of the clinic visit	Respondents self-report height and weight and the CDC uses the measurements to calculate each respondents' BMI	Medical personnel measure respondents' height and weight to calculate BMI as part of the physical examination

Source: Centers for Disease Control and Prevention, "National Health and Nutrition Examination Survey," at http://www.cdc.gov/nchs/nhanes.htm; "Youth Risk Behavior Surveillance System," at http://www.cdc.gov/ HealthyYouth/yrbs/index.htm; "Pediatric Nutrition Surveillance System," at http://www.cdc.gov/pednss/ index.htm; Maternal and Child Health Bureau, Health Resources and Statistics Administration, "National Survey of Children's Health," at http://www.cdc.gov/pednss/index.htm.

Notes:

a. Native Hawaiian and Other Pacific Islander.

b. American Indian and Alaskan Native.

c. Participation in these surveillance systems varies from year to year; some contributors do not participate every year.

Appendix B. Overweight and Obesity by Age and Sex

Table B-1. Percentage of Children and Adolescents with High BMI, by Sex and Age, 2007-2008.

	All	Age 2-5	Age 6-11	Age12-19
All Children				
≥ 85% Percentile	31.7	21.2	35.5	34.2
≥ 95% Percentile	16.9	10.4	19.6	18.1
≥ 97% Percentile	11.9	6.9	14.5	12.5
Male				
≥ 85% Percentile	32.1	21.0	35.9	35.0
≥ 95% Percentile	17.8	10.0	21.2	19.3
≥ 97% Percentile	13.0	5.8	16.3	14.3
Female				
≥ 85% Percentile	31.3	21.4	35.2	33.3
≥ 95% Percentile	15.9	10.7	18.0	16.8
≥ 97% Percentile	10.6	8.1	12.6	10.4

Source: CRS analysis based on data from NHANES (2007-2008) as presented in Ogden C, Carroll M, and Curtin L, et al., "Prevalence of High Body Mass Index in U.S. Children and Adolescents, 2007-2008," *JAMA*, vol. 303, no. 3 (January 13, 2010), pp. 242-249.

Appendix C. Overweight and Obesity by Race/Ethnicity and Sex

Table C-1. Percentage of Children and Adolescents with High BMI Age 2 Through 19 Years, by Sex and Race/Ethnicity, 2007-2008.

	All	Non-Hispanic White	Non-Hispanic Black	All Hispanics	Mexican-American
All					
≥ 85% Percentile	31.7	29.3	35.9	38.2	38.9
≥ 95% Percentile	16.9	15.3	20.0	20.9	20.8
≥ 97% Percentile	11.9	10.5	14.9	15.2	14.9
Male					
≥ 85% Percentile	32.1	29.5	33.0	39.9	41.7
≥ 95% Percentile	17.8	15.7	17.3	24.4	24.9
≥ 97% Percentile	13.0	11.4	14.1	17.6	17.7
Female					
≥ 85% Percentile	31.3	29.2	39.0	36.4	36.1
≥ 95% Percentile	15.9	14.9	22.7	17.2	16.5
≥ 97% Percentile	10.6	9.6	15.7	12.6	11.9

Source: CRS analysis based on data from NHANES (2007-2008) as presented in Ogden C, Carroll M, and Curtin L, et al., "Prevalence of High Body Mass Index in U.S. Children and Adolescents, 2007-2008," *JAMA*, vol. 303, no. 3 (January 13, 2010), pp. 242-249.

End Notes

[1] Ogden C, Carroll M, and Curtin L, et al., "Prevalence of High Body Mass Index in U.S. Children and Adolescents, 2007-2008," *JAMA*, vol. 303, no. 3 (January 13, 2010), pp. 242-249.
In children and adolescents, obesity is defined as being at or above the 95th percentile of the age- and sex-specific body mass index (BMI); overweight is defined as being between the 85th and 94th percentiles.

[2] Dietz W, "Health Consequences of Obesity in Youth: Childhood Predictors of Adult Disease," *Pediatrics*, 1998, vol. 101, pp. 518–525.

[3] American Academy of Pediatrics, Committee on Nutrition. "Prevention of Pediatric Overweight and Obesity," *Pediatrics*, 112(2): 424-430, August 2003.

[4] Stewart ST, Cutler DM and Rosen AB. "Forecasting the Effects of Obesity and Smoking on U.S. Life Expectancy," *New England Journal of Medicine*, 361(23):2252-2260, December 3, 2009.

[5] Finkelstein E, Trogdon J, Cohen J, et al., "Annual Medical Spending Attributable to Obesity: Payer and Service-Specific Estimates," *Health Affairs*, 28(5), 2009. Mission: Readiness, Military Leaders for Kids. "Too Fat to Fight: Retired Military Leaders Want Junk Food Out of America's Schools," Mission Readiness, New York, 2010.

[6] Office of the Surgeon General, *The Surgeon General's Vision for a Healthy and Fit Nation*, Department of Health and Human Services, Rockville, MD, January 2010, http://www.surgeongeneral.gov/library/obesityvision/ obesityvision2010.pdf.

[7] White House Task Force on Childhood Obesity, *Solving the Problem of Childhood Obesity Within a Generation*, Report to the President, Washington, DC, May 2010, http://www.letsmove.gov/taskforce_childhoodobesityrpt.html.

[8] Centers for Disease Control and Prevention, *Defining Overweight and Obesity*, http://www.cdc.gov/obesity defining.html.

[9] U.S. Preventive Services Task Force. Screening for Obesity in Children and Adolescents: U.S. Preventive Services Task Force Recommendation Statement. *Pediatrics* 2010;125:361-367.

[10] A quick assessment of child and teen BMI can be found online at http://apps.nccd.cdc.gov/dnpabmi/.

[11] Mei Z, Grummer-Strawn LM, Pietrobelli A, et al., "Validity of Body Mass Index Compared with Other Body-Composition Screening Indexes for the Assessment of Body Fatness in Children and Adolescents," *American Journal of Clinical Nutrition* 2002; 978–985.

[12] Ogden C, Kuczmarski R, and Flegal K, et al., "Centers for Disease Control and Prevention 2000 Growth Charts for the United States: Improvements to the 1977 National Center for Health Statistics Version," *Pediatrics*, vol. 109 (2002), pp. 45-60.

[13] In the past, children at the 85th percentile were considered "at-risk for overweight," and those at the 95th percentile were considered "overweight." An American Medical Association expert panel recommended a change in terminology in 2007 to "overweight" for children at or above the 85th percentile and "obese" for children at or above the 95th percentile, respectively. CDC and NCHS have adopted this terminology, based on the AMA panel's recommendation. The updated terms are used in this report.

[14] National Center for Health Statistics, CDC, *National Health and Nutrition Examination Survey, 2007-2008*, Overview, Hyattsville, MD, http://www.cdc.gov/nchs/data/nhanes/nhanes_07_08/overviewbrochure_0708.pdf.

[15] CDC, *Morbidity and Mortality Weekly Report, Youth Risk Behavior Surveillance—2007*, Atlanta , GA, June 6, 2008, http://www.cdc.gov/mmwr/PDF/ss/ss5704.pdf.

[16] Polhamus B, Dalenius K, and Mackentosh H, et al., *Pediatric Nutrition Surveillance 2008 Report*, CDC, Atlanta, GA, 2009, http://www.cdc.gov/pednss/pdfs/PedNSS_2008.pdf.

[17] Majid Ezzati, Hilarie Martin, and Suzanne Skj old, et al., "Trends in National and Sate-level Obesity in the USA After Correction for Self-Report Bias: Analysis of Health Surveys," Journal of the Royal Society of Medicine, vol. 99 (2006), pp. 250-257.

[18] Ogden C, Carroll M, and Curtin L, et al., "Prevalence of High Body Mass Index in U.S. Children and Adolescents, 2007-2008," *JAMA*, vol. 303, no. 3 (January 13, 2010), pp. 242-249.

[19] Ogden C, Carroll M, "Prevalence of Obesity among Children and Adolescents, United States, Trends 1963-1965 through 2007-2008. NCHS Health E-Stat: http://www.cdc.gov/nchs/data/hestat/obesity obesity_child_07_08.htm.

[20] U.S. Department of Health and Human Services. "Healthy People 2010," 2nd ed. with Understanding and Improving Health and Objectives for Improving Health. 2 vols. Washington, DC: U.S. Government Printing Office, November 2000.

[21] Ogden C, Carroll M, "Prevalence of Obesity among Children and Adolescents, United States, Trends 1963-1965 through 2007-2008. NCHS Health E-Stat: http://www.cdc.gov/nchs/data/hestat/obesity obesity _child _07 _08.htm.

[22] Ogden, CL, Carroll MD, and Curtin LR, et al., "Prevalence of High Body Mass Index," *JAMA*, vol. 303, no. 3 (January 20, 2010), pp. 242-249.

[23] Ogden, CL, Carroll MD, and Curtin LR, et al., "Prevalence of High Body Mass Index," *JAMA*, vol. 303, no. 3 (January 20, 2010), pp. 242-249. http://www.cdc.gov/nchs/data/hestat/obesity

[24] Wang Y and Beydoun MA, "The Obesity Epidemic in the United States—Gender, Age, Socioeconomic, Racial/Ethnic, and Geographic Characteristics: A Systematic Review and Meta-Regression Analysis," *Epidemiol Rev*, vol. 29 (2007), pp. 6-28.

[25] Wang Y and Beydoun MA, "The Obesity Epidemic in the United States—Gender, Age, Socioeconomic, Racial/Ethnic, and Geographic Characteristics: A Systematic Review and Meta-Regression Analysis," *Epidemiol Rev*, vol. 29 (2007), pp. 6-28.

[26] Singh G, Siahpush M, and Kogan M, "Rising Social Inequalities in US Childhood Obesity, 2003-2007," *Ann Epidemiol*, vol. 20 (2010), pp. 40-52.

[27] Morbidity and Mortality Weekly Report, *Obesity Prevalence Among Low-Income, Preschool-Aged Children—United States, 1998-2008*, CDC, Atlanta, GA, July 24, 2009, 769-773.

[28] Centers for Disease Control and Prevention, Atlanta, GA, accessed March 19, 2010, http://www.cdc.gov/obesity childhood/causes.html.

[29] Singh G, Siahpush M, and Kogan M, "Rising Social Inequalities in U.S. Childhood Obesity, 2003-2007," *Ann Epidemiol*, vol. 20 (2010), pp. 40-52.

[30] Singh G, Siahpush M, and Kogan M, "Neighborhood Socioeconomic Conditions, Built Environments, and Childhood Obesity," *Health Affairs*, vol. 29, no. 3 (2010), pp. 503-5 12.

[31] Arenz S, Rucker R, and Koletzko B, et al., "Breastfeeding and Childhood Obesity—A Systematic Review," *Int J Obes Relat Metab Disord*, vol. 28 (2004), pp. 1247-1256.

[32] Krauss R, Winston M, and Fletcher B, et al., "Obesity: Impact on Cardiovascular Disease," *Circulation*, vol. 98 (1998), pp. 1472-1476. Dietz W, "Health Consequences of Obesity in Youth: Childhood Predictors of Adult Disease," *Pediatrics*, 1998, vol. 101, pp. 518–525.

[33] Centers for Disease Control and Prevention, Atlanta, GA, accessed March 19, 2010, http://www.cdc.gov/obesity childhood/consequences.html.

[34] Whitaker RC, Wright JA, and Pepe MS, et al., "Predicting Obesity in Young Adulthood from Childhood and Parental Obesity," *NEJM*, vol. 337, no. 13 (1997), pp. 869-73.

[35] Flegal K, Graubard B, and Williamson D, et al., "Excess Deaths Associated with Underweight, Overweight, and Obesity," *JAMA*, vol. 293, no. 15 (April 20, 2005), pp. 1861-1867.

[36] Mokdad A, Marks J, and Stroup D, et al., "Actual Causes of Death in the United States, 2000," *JAMA*, vol. 291, no. 10 (March 10, 2004), pp. 1238-1245.

[37] Franks PW, Hanson RL, and Knowler W, et al., "Childhood Obesity, Other Cardiovascular Risk Factors, and Premature Death," *NEJM*, vol. 362, no. 6 (February 11, 2010), pp. 485-93.

[38] Swartz MB, and Puhl R, "Childhood Obesity: a Societal Problem to Solve," *Obesity Reviews* 2003, vol. 4, no. 1, pp. 57–7 1.

[39] Bethell C, Simpson L, and Stumbo S, et al., "National, State, and Local Disparities in Childhood Obesity," *Health Affairs*, vol. 29, no. 3 (2010), pp. 347-356.

[40] Lynn Parker, Annina Catherine Burns, and Eduardo Sanchez, Editors, *Local Government Actions to Prevent Childhood Obesity*, Institute of Medicine, Washington, DC, September 2009.

In: Solving Childhood Obesity
Editors: Sarah J. Maier and Natalie E. Brunner
ISBN: 978-1-61209-964-4

Chapter 3

The Surgeon General's Vision for a Healthy and Fit Nation 2010

U.S. Department of Health and Human Services

Message from the Surgeon General

Our nation stands at a crossroads. Today's epidemic of overweight and obesity threatens the historic progress we have made in increasing American's quality and years of healthy life. Two-third of adults[1] and nearly one in three children are overweight or obese.[2] In addition, many racial and ethnic groups and geographic regions of the United States are disproportionately affected.[3] The sobering impact of these numbers is reflected in the nation's concurrent epidemics of diabetes, heart disease, and other chronic diseases. If we do not reverse these trends, researchers warn that many of our children—our most precious resource—will be seriously afflicted in early adulthood with medical conditions such as diabetes and heart disease. This future is unacceptable. I ask you to join me in combating this crisis.

Every one of us has an important role to play in the prevention and control of obesity. Mothers, fathers, teachers, business executives, child care professionals, clinicians, politicians, and government and community leaders—we must all commit to changes that promote the health and wellness of our families and communities. As a nation, we must create neighborhood communities that are focused on healthy nutrition and regular physical activity, where the healthiest choices are accessible for all citizens. Children should be having fun and playing in environments that provide parks, recreational facilities, community centers, and walking and bike paths. Healthy foods should be affordable and accessible. Increased consumer knowledge and awareness about healthy nutrition and physical activity will foster a growing demand for healthy food products and exercise options, dramatically influencing marketing trends.

Hospitals, work sites, and communities should make it easy for mothers to initiate and sustain breastfeeding as this practice has been shown to prevent childhood obesity. Working together, we will create an environment that promotes and facilitates healthy choices for all Americans. And we will live longer and healthier lives.

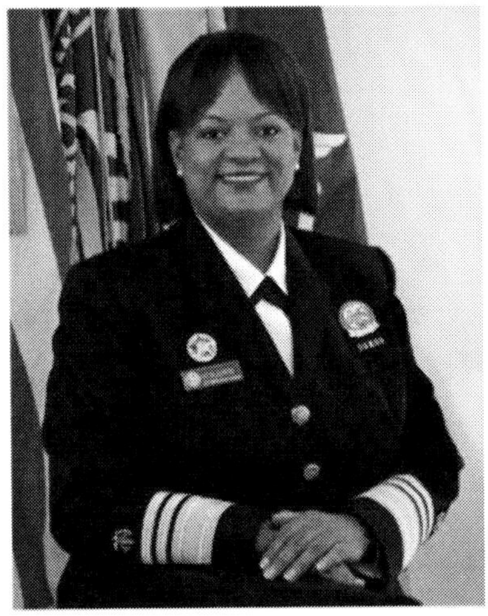

In the 2001 *Surgeon General's Call to Action to Prevent and Decrease Overweight and Obesity*, former Surgeon General David Satcher, MD, PhD, warned us of the negative effects of the increasing weight of our citizens and outlined a public health response to reverse the trend.[4] I plan to strengthen and expand this blueprint for action created by my predecessor. Although we have made some strides since 2001, the prevalence of obesity, obesity-related diseases, and premature death remains too high.

I am calling on all Americans to join me in a national grassroots effort to reverse this trend. My plan includes showing people how to choose nutritious food, add more physical activity to their daily lives, and manage the stress that so often derails their best efforts at developing healthy habits. I envision men, women, and children who are mentally and physically fit to live their lives to the fullest. The real goal is not just a number on a scale, but optimal health for all Americans at every stage of life. To achieve this goal, we must all work together to share resources, educate our citizens, and partner with business and government leaders to find creative solutions in our neighborhoods, towns, and cities from coast to coast. Together, we can become a nation committed to become healthy and fit.

Regina M. Benjamin, MD, MBA
VADM, USPHS
Surgeon General

BACKGROUND ON OBESITY

Obesity poses a major public health challenge. Each year, obesity contributes to an estimated 112,000 preventable deaths.[5] Obese adults are at increased risk for many serious health conditions, including high blood pressure, high cholesterol, type 2 diabetes and its complications, coronary heart disease, stroke, gallbladder disease, osteoarthritis, sleep apnea, and respiratory problems, as well as endometrial, breast, prostate, and colon cancers.[6] Children with a high body mass index (BMI), an indicator of excess body weight, are more likely than those with a normal BMI to have insulin resistance[7](which can lead to diabetes), high blood pressure, and unhealthy levels of fats and other lipids. Furthermore, obese children often become obese adults; some studies have found that even 2- to 5- year-olds with a high BMI are likely to become obese adults.[8] Besides suffering from physical illnesses, obese adults and children also may experience social stigmatization and discrimination, as well as psychological problems.

In recent decades, the prevalence of obesity has increased dramatically in the United States, tripling among children and doubling among adults.[1-2,9-10] This epidemic increase is the result of specific changes in our environment and behaviors in susceptible people. High-calorie, good-tasting, and inexpensive foods have become widely available and are heavily advertised. Portion sizes have increased,[11] and we are eating out more frequently.[12] Our children drink more sugar-sweetened beverages than they did in the past, and they are drinking fewer beverages such as water or low or non- fat milk[13] that are healthier for growing minds and bodies.

However, dietary changes are not completely responsible for the epidemic.

Widespread adoption of multiple technological innovations in the home, workplace, and schools has reduced our daily physical activity. Similarly, the car-dependent design of our communities has made it much harder for our children to walk to school—and much harder for us to shop and do other errands entirely on foot or by bicycle. On top of these changes, many of our nation's schools have cut back or eliminated recess and physical education programs.[14]

This document highlights the trends, health consequences, and causes related to the obesity epidemic. Given the multiple social changes behind the epidemic, this brief also proposes health- promoting actions that can be taken by multiple sectors of society.

Trends

The prevalence of obesity changed relatively little during the 1960s and 1970s, but it increased sharply over the ensuing decades—from 13.4% in 1980 to 34.3% in 2008 among adults and from 5% to 17% among children during the same period.[1-2,9- 10] The prevalence of extreme obesity also increased during 1976–1980 and 2007–2008, and approximately 6% of U.S. adults now have a BMI of 40 kg/m2 or higher.[15]

The United States is not alone in experiencing an obesity epidemic. Similar increases in the prevalence of obesity have been reported in developed countries such as England and in countries where obesity was formerly rare.[16-17] For example, the prevalence in China among preschool-aged children living in urban areas has increased eightfold—from 1.5% in 1989 to 12.6% in 1997.[18]

Disparities

The burden of obesity is disproportionately borne by some racial and ethnic groups. For example, among 40- to 59-year-old women, about 52% of non-Hispanic blacks and 47% of Hispanics are obese; for non-Hispanic whites, the prevalence is 36%.[19] These differences also are seen among children and teenagers. For example, obesity is much more common among non-Hispanic black teenagers (29%) than among Hispanic teenagers (17.5%) or non-Hispanic white teenagers (14.5%). [19]

The burden of obesity and the severity of related health conditions vary among different population groups. While obesity is a public health crisis within the general population, it is even more prevalent in persons with mental illness [20-21] with some reports indicating 83% of people with serious mental illness being overweight or obese.[22] This puts people with mental disorders in double jeopardy. Not only are they dealing with a mental disorder that often leads to social isolation, a sedentary lifestyle and physical inactivity – all risk factors for obesity - but they are also vulnerable to the chronic diseases associated with being overweight, mood instability and low self-esteem.[23] People with serious mental illness have shortened life-spans, on average living only until 53 years of age.[24] Their deaths are not brought on by their mental illness, but rather from other chronic health conditions, including obesity. Many people are not aware that rapid weight gain is one of the most common and alarming side effects of psychiatric medications for both children and adults.[25] Youth aged 4 to 19 being treated with antipsychotic medications gained more than 7% of their total body weight in 12 weeks.[26] Clearly persons with mental illness are a vulnerable population at high-risk for obesity and obesity- related disorders.

Measuring Overweight and Obesity

Obesity is generally defined as excess body fat. However, since excess body fat is difficult to measure directly, obesity is often defined as excess body weight as measured by BMI. BMI, which is calculated as weight in kilograms divided by height in meters squared, is used to express weight adjusted for height. Although BMI has limitations as a measure,[27] it has been a useful indicator of overweight and obesity. For example, several studies have found that adults with a high BMI are at increased risk for various diseases[6] and children who have a high BMI are likely to have relatively high levels of body fatness.[28] Adults who have a BMI of 25.0 to 29.9 are considered to be overweight, those with a BMI ≥30 are considered obese, and those with a BMI ≥ 40 are considered extremely obese.[6,29]

In overweight and obese adults and children, other health risk factors (such as blood pressure, blood sugar, and blood fats) should be assessed, as recommended by published guidelines. Because excess body fatness in the abdomen can be a marker for increased health risk even at a lower BMI, measurement of waist circumference is recommended in overweight and obese adults.[30] BMI does not distinguish between lean tissue and body fat, and some growing children or athletic children and adults will have a BMI in the overweight or obese range without having an excess of body fat.[31] However, most children and adults with a BMI in the range considered obese will also have excess body fat.

Underweight	≤ 18.5
Healthy Weight	18.5-24.9
Overweight	25-29.9
Obese	≥ 30

Figure 1. Adult BMI Classification.

Underweight	≤ 5th percentile
Healthy Weight	5th to the 85th percentile
Overweight	85th to the 95th percentile
Obese	≥ 95th percentile

*BMI for Age Percentile [Age 2-19]

Figure 2. Children BMI Classification.

Assessing if a child is at a healthy weight is complex. While BMI is often utilized, clinical assessment and other markers should be considered when determining a child's overall health and development. Among children, the marked BMI changes that occur with growth and development make it necessary to specify a high BMI relative to children of the same sex and age. The 2000 CDC growth charts are[32] used for this purpose in the United States. Children and adolescents with a BMI at or above the sex-and age-specific 95th percentile of this reference population are often considered obese, and those with a BMI between the 85th and 94th percentiles are often considered overweight.[33] Although these cut points are not diagnostic criteria, elevated BMI among children most often indicates increased risk for future adverse health outcomes and/or development of disease.

Health Consequences

Obesity in early life has been found to increase the risk for various diseases in adulthood, including diabetes and heart disease, in part because obese children are likely to become obese adults.[34-35] Several studies also have found short-term effects of excess weight during childhood—for example, high BMI levels among children and teenagers are associated with childhood development of atherosclerosis.[36-38]

The growing U.S. obesity epidemic is reflected in the tripling, since 1980, of the number of Americans who have diabetes.[39] Approximately 8% of U.S. adults have type 2 diabetes,[40] a disease that increases the risk for cardiovascular disease, stroke, kidney disease, blindness, lower- limb amputation and other problems. Obesity is the most important risk factor for type 2 diabetes.[41] Although type 2 diabetes has traditionally been viewed as developing among middle-aged (or older) adults, type 2 diabetes is now occurring in early life.[42] Although the rate of type 2 diabetes in children has increased, it is very low[42] (one quarter of 1 percent), but more than 75% of children and adolescents with type 2 diabetes are obese.[43-44] The poor glycemic control of many adolescents with type 2 diabetes,[45] along with the increased duration of diabetes diagnosed in early life, may increase the risk of subsequent complications.

Causes of Obesity

In addition to consuming too many calories and not getting enough physical activity, genes, metabolism, behavior, environment, and culture can also play a role in causing people to be overweight and obese. Identifying determinants of and supporting changes in behaviors and in the environment are likely to be the most effective actions to combat obesity. Key modifiable risk factors are physical activity, sedentary behavior and diet. Physical activity plays several important roles in the prevention and control of obesity, and it is essential for health at any weight. Increased physical activity and decreased sedentary behavior are associated with lower rates of obesity, and it reduces the risk for many of the diseases associated with obesity, such as diabetes and heart disease.

A healthy diet is also important. Beginning early in life, breastfeeding is a relatively short-term intervention which has significant long-term potential for maintaining a lower BMI.[46] At any stage of life, increased consumption of excess calories from fats and added sugars in foods that are energy dense, such as fast food, is associated with obesity. These foods are relatively higher in calories than nutrients that are needed for health. Sugar-sweetened beverages, such as soda, contribute to excess calorie intake from added sugars or displace more nutritious foods in the diet. Some evidence suggests that the body may not compensate for the calories consumed with these beverages.[47] In contrast, consumption of fruits and vegetables in place of high calorie foods may reduce the risk for obesity and help sustain weight loss because the body's sense of fullness at meals is partly regulated by volume. Fruits and vegetables contain few calories and are bulky foods, so they have a low caloric density and are more filling than fast foods.

The amount of time spent watching television is another association with obesity in both children and adults. The association with obesity may be mediated in part by the effects of television time on food consumption. The more time children spend watching television, the more likely they are to eat while doing so and the more likely they are to eat the high-calorie foods that are heavily advertised on television.[48]

Stress is another contributing factor to overweight and obesity. Studies have shown chronic stress adversely affects blood pressure and cholesterol and may lead persons to increase their caloric intake.[49] Furthermore stress may limit people's motivation and ability to adopt positive weight-related behaviors.[50]

Opportunities for Prevention

Interventions to prevent obesity should focus not only on personal behaviors and biological traits, but also on characteristics of the social and physical environments that offer or limit opportunities for positive health outcomes. Critical opportunities for interventions can occur in multiple settings: home, child care, school, work place, health care, and community.

Individual Healthy Choices and Healthy Home Environments

As a society, we have to begin to change our habits one healthy choice at a time. Change starts with the individual choices we as Americans make each day for ourselves and those around us. Balancing good nutrition and physical activity while managing daily stressors is always a challenge, but one that can be achieved. Finding time to shop for and prepare healthy meals after work and between family activities requires planning. Stress and a lack of available healthy and affordable foods are some of the reasons why many people turn to fast food as a regular source for meals. Eating excess calories contributes to obesity, but so does watching too much television48] and sitting for hours in front of a computer.

This fact is especially true for children and teenagers. Technological advancements have made our lives more convenient—but also more sedentary. Research shows that leading an inactive life not only increases the risk of becoming overweight or obese, but also contributes to an increased risk for disease and disability.[51]

The good news is that we can overcome these challenges—and the reward is the creation of a healthy and fit nation. Healthy choices include:[51-53]

- Reducing consumption of sodas and juices with added sugars.
- Reducing consumption of energy dense foods that primarily contain added sugars or solid fats.
- Eating more fruits, vegetables, whole grains, and lean proteins.
- Controlling your portions.
- Drinking more water.
- Choosing low-fat or non-fat dairy products.
- Limiting television viewing time and consider keeping televisions out of children's rooms.
- Becoming more physically active throughout the day.
- Breastfeeding exclusively to 6 months.

Creating a Healthy Home Environment

As adults, we need to help our children get off to a good start. The earliest risks for childhood obesity begin during pregnancy. Excess weight gain, diabetes, and smoking during pregnancy are not just health risks for the mother—they also put children at risk for obesity early in life. Keeping pregnancy weight gain within recommended limits will help prevent diabetes in the mother. Stopping cigarette smoking and abstaining from alcohol and drug use will protect the health of the mother and the baby.

The earliest decisions regarding food, activity, and television viewing occur in the home. Parents and other caregivers play a key role in making good choices for themselves and their loved one. Children and teenagers look to their mothers and fathers and other caregivers to model healthy lifestyle habits, and adults need to teach by example. In some households, several generations may live together or have responsibility for children at different times during the day. This sharing of duties requires coordination and consistency in activities and habits related to food shopping and preparation, access to physical activity, and limits on television and computer use.

Both young children and teenagers learn from the choices they see adults make. One way to help children learn is to involve all family members in family-based physical activities and in planning, shopping for, and preparing meals. These activities provide both an education in healthy nutrition and exercise, as well as a critical foundation for how to make healthy lifestyle choices.

Healthy Food Choices

The first decision that parents make about what to feed their child occurs during pregnancy. After the baby is born, mothers should breastfeed whenever possible because it provides the highest quality of nutrition and helps to prevent early childhood obesity.[46] By age 2, children should be drinking low-fat or non-fat milk. As parents, we are in charge of the foods we provide to our children. Creativity with food preparation can often solve the problems presented by picky eaters. Adults also should offer children small portions and show them how to eat slowly and enjoy their meal.

Healthy Teenagers

The teenage years present unique challenges. Adolescence is a time of vulnerability to the development of psychiatric disorders, including eating disorders, depression, drug and alcohol abuse. Adolescent boys and girls are subjected to significant peer pressure related to eating and exercise, and most school systems provide limited opportunities for physical activity. Teenagers often drink more carbonated and caffeinated beverages and eat more fast foods. These multiple stresses and unhealthy habits make teenagers particularly vulnerable to becoming sedentary, overweight, and obese. An obese teenager has a greater than 70% risk of becoming an obese adult.[34] Parents should guide their teenagers to become fit and healthy adults while being cautious not to trigger unhealthy eating behaviors or eating disorders.

Physical Activity

Scheduling time for the recommended levels of physical activity is essential to overall health. Physical activity can help control weight, reduce risk for many diseases (heart disease and some cancers), strengthen your bones and muscles, improve your mental health, and increase your chances of living longer.[51]

Adults should do at least 150 minutes of moderate-intensity physical activity per week.[51] Aerobic activity such as brisk walking or general gardening should be done in episodes of at least 10 minutes and preferably should be spread throughout the week. For children and teenagers, the recommendation is for 1 hour of daily physical activity that includes vigorous activities and activities that strengthen their bones.[51]

Making physical activities fun can affect how children and teenagers respond to changes in their routine. Programmed, repetitious exercise may work for adults, but it rarely works for children. Look for ways to add physical activity throughout the day. When possible, parents should walk with children to and from school, and children should have scheduled time to play. Because safety is a real concern in many neighborhoods, citizens should talk with their local elected officials and members of law enforcement to find ways to improve safety so everyone can walk or play outdoors.

Television and Computer Use

In recent years, we have witnessed an explosion of technological advances in televisions, home entertainment centers, computers, and video game players. A new report released in 2010[54] found that nearly two-thirds of kids aged 8 - 18 say the TV is usually on during meals and nearly half report the TV is left on "most of the time" in their home. Seven in ten young people have a TV in their bedroom and 50% also have a console video game player in their room. Overall, 8-18 year-olds spend over 7 hours per day using entertainment media (TV, video games, computers) amounting to more than 53 hours a week.

The hours that adults, teenagers, and children are spending in front of a television or computer screen contribute to their sedentary lifestyle and increase their risk for obesity. In particular, the more time children spend watching television, the more likely they are to eat while doing so and the more likely they are to eat the high-calorie food that are heavily advertised to both adults and children.[55]

Most parents either do not set limitations on screen time or don't enforce them. Studies have shown that when parents establish rules and implement them, screen time declines by 2 hours per day, leaving opportunities for more physical activity. Parents need to be role models by limiting their own television time and spending more time with their children.

Creating Healthy Child Care Settings

Early childhood settings, including child care and early childhood education programs, affect the lives of millions of U.S. children. In 2005, 61% of children aged 0–6 years who were not yet in kindergarten (about 12 million children) received some form of child care on a regular basis from someone other than their parents.[56] Child care programs should identify and implement approaches that reflect expert recommendations on physical activity, screen time limitations, good nutrition, and healthy sleep practices. Early childhood providers, like parents, should model healthy lifestyle behaviors and teach children how to make healthy choices. They also should reach out to parents to encourage them to practice and promote healthy habits at home.

To choose a healthy child care environment, parents should:

- Ask childcare providers about their approach to promoting healthy lifestyles for children.
- Visit the setting to see how childcare providers model and teach physical activity, good nutrition, and healthy sleep practices.
- Ask childcare providers how they keep parents informed about what they can do at home to support their child's physical activity, good nutrition, and healthy sleep practices.
- Ask childcare providers about their support of breastfeeding, breast milk storage and handling.

Child care providers should:

- Identify and use resources that recommend effective approaches to promoting physical activity, good nutrition, and healthy sleep in early childhood settings.
- Establish and post policies, procedures, and practices that support these approaches in ways that respect local communities and cultures.
- Stay current in these approaches through required regular training.
- Educate and involve parents in trainings and other activities.

State regulations regarding physical activity, nutrition, and screen time vary greatly among child care settings by state and type (e.g., Head Start, center-based child care, family-based child care). Standardized national goals for early child care—especially ones related to healthy weight— would improve the quality of early childhood settings and give childcare providers and parents a foundation to improve their knowledge and skills to support these goals.

For example, recommended policies that can help child care programs support healthy weight for young children include the following:

- Require 60 minutes of a mix of structured and unstructured daily physical activity.
- Establish nutrition requirements in child care by using national recommendations such as the *Dietary G uidelines for Americans*.
- Use a structured approach to training child care providers how to promote physical activity and good nutrition and how to educate and involve parents in these activities.
- Give parents materials that reinforce the practices of child care settings that promote physical activity and good nutrition and limit screen time.

Creating Healthy Schools

Schools play a pivotal role in preventing obesity among children and teenagers. Each school day provides multiple opportunities for students to learn about health and practice healthy behaviors that affect weight, including physical activity and good nutrition. Well-designed school programs can promote physical activity and healthy eating, reduce the rate of overweight and obesity among children and teenagers, and improve academic achievement.[57-64]

To ensure that nutrition and physical activity programs are effective, school administrations need physical education specialists, health education specialists, and certified food service staff. Schools should encourage and reinforce healthy dietary behaviors by providing nutritious and appealing foods and beverages in all venues accessible to students, including the cafeteria, vending machines, school stores, and concession stands. A substantial percentage of students' recommended physical activity can be provided through a comprehensive school-based physical activity program that includes high-quality physical education, recess and other physical activity breaks, intramurals and physical activity clubs, interscholastic sports, and walk- and biketo-school initiatives.[65-66]

High-quality physical education gives young people a chance to learn the skills needed to establish and maintain physically active lifestyles throughout their lives. States and local school districts set requirements for physical activity levels.

In 2006, few schools provided daily physical education or its equivalent for the entire school year to all students.[67] Nationwide, only 30% of high school students attended physical education classes 5 days in an average school week, compared with 42% in 1991.[68]

To help students develop healthy habits, schools should have comprehensive wellness plans that include:

- An active school health council to guide health-related policy decisions.
- A planned and sequential health education curriculum for pre-kindergarten through grade 12. This curriculum should be based on national standards and address a clear set of behavioral outcomes that empower students to make healthy dietary choices and meet physical activity recommendations.
- A school and school workplace wellness policy that includes teachers and other school employees to model healthy behaviors.
- A comprehensive professional development and credentialing program for staff that addresses health education, physical education, food service, and health services.
- Partnerships with parent-teacher organizations, families, and community members to support healthy eating and physical activity policies and programs.

To promote healthy nutrition, schools should:

- Establish nutrition standards that promote healthy nutritious foods.
- Ensure availability of appealing, healthy food options that that enable students to comply with recommendations in the U.S. Dietary Guidelines for Americans, including fresh fruits and vegetables, whole grains, and lean proteins.
- Use presentation, marketing, and education techniques to encourage students to eat more fruits and vegetables, whole grains, and lean proteins and to drink more water and low-fat or non-fat beverages.
- Make sure water is available throughout the school setting.
- Limit amounts of high calorie snack options, including beverages in vending machines.

To promote physical activity, school systems should:

- Require daily physical education for students in pre-kindergarten through grade 12, allowing 150 minutes per week for elementary schools and 225 minutes per week for secondary schools.
- Require and implement a planned and sequential physical education curriculum for pre-kindergarten through grade 12 that is based on national standards.
- Require at least 20 minutes daily recess for all students in elementary schools.
- Offer students opportunities to participate in intramural physical activity programs during after-school hours.

- Implement and promote walk- and biketo-school programs.
- Establish joint use agreements with local government agencies to allow use of school facilities for physical activity programs offered by the school or community-based organizations outside of school hours.

Creating Healthy Work Sites

The majority of the 140 million men and women who are employed in the United States spend a significant amount of time each week at their work site. Wellness programs in the workplace are an effective way to support people's efforts to achieve and maintain a healthy weight.[69] Because obesity reduces worker productivity [70-71] and increases health care costs, employers are becoming more aware of the need to address risk factors for poor nutrition and physical inactivity through workplace initiatives.

Research has shown that health promotion programs in the workplace can be cost effective and well worth the ongoing costs of implementing these programs.[72-75] Because the health and productivity of an employer's workforce is affected by the vitality of the communities in which employees reside, businesses will benefit from being actively involved in health promotion efforts within their communities.[76]

To create healthy work sites, employers can:

- Establish and promote creative work site wellness programs, ask employees to be wellness champions, and set up ongoing employee challenges.
- Support employees who want to breastfeed by providing written policies and designated private, clean spaces for breastfeeding or expressing milk.
- Create a culture of wellness by integrating messages about the benefits of physical activity and healthy eating into the workplace.
- Provide opportunities and incentives for physical activity through onsite facilities, group classes or personal training, outdoor exercise areas, walking paths, and stairwell programs.
- Make healthy food and beverage available and affordable in the workplace.
- Become active partners in the health promotion efforts of local community groups, such as community coalitions and task forces.
- Sponsor community health events.
- Help develop government policy and legislative initiatives that support employee wellness programs.
- Provide health benefits that offer employees and their dependents coverage for obesity-related services and programs.

Mobilizing the Medical Community

In 2002, Americans made an estimated 166 million visits to medical offices.[77] People access the health care system through multiple channels, and medical care settings are an important avenue for preventing and controlling overweight and obesity. Clinicians are often the most trusted source of health information and can be powerful role models for healthy lifestyle habits.

Clinicians should make it a priority to teach their patients about the importance of achieving and maintaining a healthier body weight, becoming more physically active, selecting healthier food options and managing stress. They should provide comprehensive resources to help patients make healthy lifestyle choices. These resources should include in-office access or referrals to registered dietitians, health educators, counselors, psychologists, and fitness professionals, as well as to links to community resources.[78]

To help their patients make healthy lifestyle choices, clinicians should:

- Measure patients' BMI and explain the connection between BMI and increased risk for disease and disability.
- Record patients' physical activity levels and stress the importance of consistent exercise and daily physical activity.
- Assess and record information on patients' dietary patterns.
- Use terms that are appropriate for families and children to define healthy weight and BMI and explain how to achieve this goal.
- Work as a team to provide a comprehensive assessment and learning experience for each patient.
- Ensure that patients are referred to resources (both internal and external) that will help them meet their psychological, nutritional, and physical activity needs
- Promote awareness about the connection between mental and addiction disorders and obesity.
- For treatment of people with severe mental illness who are at risk for overweight or obesity, consider medications that are more weight neutral.

To support clinicians and their staff, the health care system should:

- Encourage clinicians and their staff to practice healthy lifestyle behaviors and be role models for their patients.
- Use best practice guidelines to teach health professional students and clinicians how to counsel patients on effective ways to achieve and maintain healthy lifestyle habits.
- Promote effective prenatal counseling about maternal weight gain, breastfeeding, the relationship between obesity and diabetes, and the need to avoid alcohol, tobacco, and drug use during pregnancy.
- Help clinicians and their staff advocate for community strategies that improve nutrition and physical activity resources for their patients.
- Promote innovative ways that clinicians and their staff can advocate for policy changes at local, state, and federal levels that will make it easier for their patients to adopt and sustain healthy habits.

Improving Our Communities

Americans need to live and work in environments that help them practice healthy behaviors. The social, cultural, physical, and economic foundations of a community are important factors in its ability to support a healthy lifestyle for its citizens. For example, government and private organizations should pool their resources to increase access to healthy foods—such as ensuring that all neighborhoods, especially in low-income areas, have full-service and safe options for physical activities, such as walking and bike paths, sidewalks, and parks.

To reverse the obesity epidemic, every neighborhood and community should become actively involved in grassroots efforts to create healthier environments for all citizens, from infants to older adults. Individuals and groups of private citizens should work closely with community leaders to make the changes needed to support healthy lifestyles.

To help lead our nation toward healthy eating and active living, The Centers for Disease Control and Prevention has recommended the following strategies:[79]

- Increase availability of healthy, affordable food and beverage choices in public service venues.
- Improve geographic availability of supermarkets in underserved areas.
- Improve access to fresh fruits and vegetables by providing incentives for the production, distribution, and procurement of foods from local farms.
- Limit advertisements of less-healthy foods and beverages.
- Increase support for breastfeeding.
- Promote exclusive breastfeeding and worksite accommodations to express human milk.
- Improve access to outdoor recreational facilities.
- Build or enhance infrastructures to support more walking and bicycling.
- Support locating schools within easy walking distance of residential areas.
- Improve access to public transportation.
- Support mixed-use development.
- Enhance personal and traffic safety in areas where people are or could be physically active.
- Participate in community coalitions or partnerships to address obesity.

Community coalitions across the United States are working with their leaders, advocating for change, and seeing real results. All communities across the country should have community coalitions that focus on the health and wellness of their citizens. The most effective coalitions include representation from all sectors— businesses, clinicians, schools, academia, government, and the faith community. These groups work together to assess the physical and social community, develop a plan when change is needed, and take action. History has shown that grassroots movements can make positive changes in their communities.

Closing Statement and Charge from the Surgeon General

To stop the obesity epidemic in this country, we must remember that Americans will be more likely to change their behavior if they have a meaningful reward—something more than just reaching a certain weight or BMI measurement. The real reward has to be something that people can feel and enjoy and celebrate. That reward is invigorating, energizing, joyous health. It is a level of health that allows people to embrace each day and live their lives to the fullest— without disease, disability, or lost productivity.

Good nutrition, regular physical activity, and stress management significantly contribute to achieving optimal health. By practicing these healthy lifestyle behaviors, excess weight is prevented, weight loss is sustained, and strength and endurance are achieved. This is the reward we need to communicate to the American public. We must help our communities make the important and life-saving connection between being healthy, fit and living well.

We are indeed at a crossroads. The "old normal" was to stress the importance of attaining recommended numbers for weight and BMI. Although these numbers are important measures of disease and disability, the total picture is much bigger. It involves the creation of a "new normal"—an emphasis on achieving an optimal level of health and well-being. People want to live long and live well, and they are making their voices heard across this nation. Today's obesity epidemic calls for committed, compassionate citizens to mobilize and demand the health and well-being they so richly deserve. I have heard this call to arms, and I am honored to do everything in my power to help Americans live long and live well.

Acknowledgments

The Surgeon General's Vision for a Healthy and Fit Nation was developed by the Office of the Surgeon General. Critical scientific oversight and writing support was provided by the Centers for Disease Control and Prevention (CDC) Division of Nutrition, Physical Activity, and Obesity. Data and analysis was provided by the (CDC) National Center for Health Statistics. Substantial scientific input was also provided by the National Institute of Diabetes and Digestive and Kidney Diseases. Technical and editorial support was also provided by numerous U.S. Department of Health and Human Services subject matter experts.

References

[1] Flegal, KM; Carroll, MD; Ogden, CL; Curtin, LR. Prevalence and trends in obesity among US adults, 1999-2008. *JAMA*. 2010, Jan 20, 303(3), 235-41. Epub 2010 Jan 13.

[2] Ogden, CL; Carroll, MD; Curtin, LR; Lamb, MM; Flegal, KM. Prevalence of high body mass index in US children and adolescents, 2007-2008, *JAMA*. 2010, Jan 20, 303(3), 242-9. Epub 2010 Jan 13.

[3] Center for Disease Control. U.S. Obesity Trends. Trends by State 1985-2008. Available at http://www.cdc.gov/obesity. Accessed: January 19, 2010.

[4] U.S. Department of Health and Human Services. The Surgeon General's Call to action to prevent and decrease overweight and obesity. (Rockville, MD): U.S. Department of

Health and Human Services, Public Health Service, Office of the Surgeon General; (2001). Available from: U.S. GPO, Washington.

[5] Flegal, KM; Graubard, BI; Williamson, DF; Gail, MH. Excess deaths associated with underweight, overweight, and obesity. *JAMA*, 2005, Apr 20, 293(15), 1861-7.

[6] Clinical Guidelines on the Identification, Evaluation, and Treatment of Overweight and Obesity in Adults--The Evidence Report. National Institutes of Health. *Obes Res*, 1998, Sep;6 Suppl 2, 51S-209S.

[7] Nathan, BM; Moran, A. Metabolic complications of obesity in childhood and adolescence: more than just diabetes. *Curr Opin Endocrinol Diabetes Obes*, 2008, Feb, 15(1), 21-9.

[8] Freedman, DS; Kettel, L; Serdula, MK; Dietz, WH; Srinivasan, SR; Berenson, GS. The Relation of Childhood BMI to Adult Adiposity: The Bogalusa Heart Study. *Pediactrics*, 2005, 115, 22-27.

[9] Flegal, KM; Carroll, MD; Ogden, CL; Johnson, CL. Prevalence and trends in obesity among US adults, 1999-2000, *JAMA*, 2002, Oct 9; 288(14), 1723-7.

[10] Ogden, CL; Flegal, KM; Carroll, MD; Johnson, CL. Prevalence and trends in overweight among US children and adolescents, 1999-2000, *JAMA* 2002, Oct 9, 288(14), 1728-32.

[11] Nielsen, SJ; Popkin, BM. Patterns and trends in food portion sizes, 1977-1998, *JAMA* 2003, Jan 22, 289(4), 450-3.

[12] Nielsen, SJ; Siega-Riz, AM; Popkin, BM. Trends in energy intake in U.S. between 1977 and 1996: similar shifts seen across age groups. *Obes Res* 2002 May; 10(5), 370-8.

[13] Nielsen, SJ; Popkin, BM. Changes in beverage intake between 1977 and 2001. *Am J Prev Med*, 2004, Oct; 27(3), 205-10.

[14] Sindelar, R. Recess: Is It Needed in the 21st Century? Early Childhood and Parenting (ECAP) Collaborative at the University of Illinois at Urbana-Champaign. July 2004. Available at http://ceep.crc.uiuc.edu/poptopics/recess.htm

[15] CDC. Prevalence of overweight, obesity, and extreme obesity among adults: United States, Trends 1976--80 through 2005-2006. Hyattsville, MD: US Department of Health and Human Services, National Center for Health Statistics, CDC; 2008.

[16] Rennie, KL; Jebb, SA. Prevalence of obesity in Great Britain. *Obes Rev*, 2005, Feb, 6(1), 11-2.

[17] Stamatakis, E; Primatesta, P; Chinn, S; Rona, R; Falascheti, E. Overweight and obesity trends from 1974 to 2003 in English children: what is the role of socioeconomic factors? *Arch Dis Child*, 2005, Oct; 90(10), 999-1004.

[18] Luo, J; Hu, FB. Time trends of obesity in preschool children in China from 1989 to 1997. *Int J Obes Relat Metab Disord*, 2002, Apr, 26(4), 553-8.

[19] Differences in Prevalence of Obesity Among Black, White, and Hispanic Adults-United States, 2006-2008, *MMWR* July 17, 2009/58(27), 740-744.

[20] Holt, R; Peveler, R. Obesity, Serious Mental Illness and Antipsychotic Drugs, Diabetes, *Obesity and Metabolism*, 2009, 11(7), 665-679.

[21] National Association of State Mental Health Program Directors. Obesity and Prevention Strategies for Individuals with Serious Mental Illness, Technical Report. 2008.

[22] Hoffmann, V; Ahl, J; Meyers, A; Schuh, L; Shults, K; Collins, D; Jensen, L. Wellness Intervention for Patients with Serious and Persistent Mental Illness, *Journal of Clinical*

Psychiatry, 2005, 66(12), 1576-1579.
[23] McIntyre, R; McElroy, S; Konarski, J; Soczynska, J; Bottas, Al, Castel, S; Wilkins, K; Kennedy, S. Substance Use Disorders and Overweight/Obesity in Bipolar Disorder: Preliminary Evidence for Competing Addictions, *Journal of Clinical Psychiatry*, 2007, 68, 1352-1357.
[24] National Association of State Mental Health Program Directors. Obesity and Prevention Strategies for Individuals with Serious Mental Illness, *Technical Report,* 2008.
[25] Simon, G; Von Korff, M; Saunders, K; Miglioretti, D; Crane, P. Van Belle, G, Kessler, R. Association Between Obesity and Psychiatric Disorders in the U.S Adult Population. *Archives of General Psychiatry*, 2006, 63(7), 824-830.
[26] Varley, C; McClellan, J. Implications of Marked Weight Gain Associated with Atypical Antipsychotic Medications in Children and Adolescents. *Journal of the American Medical Association*, 2009, 302(16), 1811-1812.
[27] Prentice, AM; Jebb, SA. Beyond body mass index. *Obes Rev*, 2001, Aug, 2(3), 141-7.
[28] Freedman, DS; Wang, J; Thornton, JC; Mei, Z; Sopher, AB; Pierson, RN; Jr, et al. Classification of body fatness by body mass index-for-age categories among children. *Arch Pediatr Adolesc Med*, 2009, Sep;163(9), 805-11.
[29] U.S. Department of Health and Human Services and U.S. Department of Agriculture. Dietary Guidelines for Americans, 2005. 6th ed. Washington, DC: U.S. Government Printing Office; 200.
[30] Clinical Guidelines on the Identification, Evaluation, and Treatment of Overweight and Obesity in Adults: The Evidence Report http://www.nhlbi.nih.gov/guidelines ob_gdlns.htm
[31] Romero-Corral, A; Montori, VM; Somers, VK; Korinek, J; Thomas, RJ; Allison, TG; Mookadam, F; Lopez-Jimenez, F. Association of bodyweight with total mortality and with cardiovascular events in coronary artery disease: a systematic review of cohort studies. *The Lancet*, 2006, 368 (9536), 666–678.
[32] Kuczmarski, RJ; Ogden, CL; Guo, SS; Grummer-Strawn, LM; Flegal, KM; Mei, Z; et al. 2000 CDC Growth Charts for the United States: methods and development. *Vital Health Stat*, 11, 2002, May;(246), 1-190.
[33] Krebs, NF; Himes, JH; Jacobson, D; Nicklas, TA; Guilday, P; Styne, D. Assessment of child and adolescent overweight and obesity. *Pediatrics*, 2007, Dec, 120 Suppl 4, S193-S228.
[34] RC; Wright, JA; Pepe, MS; Seidel, KD; Dietz, WH. Predicting obesity in young adulthood from childhood and parental obesity. *N Engl J Med,* 1997, 37(13), 869–873.
[35] Serdula, MK; Ivery, D; Coates, RJ; Freedman, DS; Williamson, DF; Byers, T. Do obese children become obese adults? A review of the literature. *Prev Med,* 1993, 22, 167-177.
[36] Dietz, W. Health consequences of obesity in youth: Childhood predictors of adult disease. *Pediatrics,* 1998, 101, 518–525.
[37] Esposito, L; Fisher, JO; Mennella, JA; Hoelscher, DM; Huang, TT. Developmental perspectives on nutrition and obesity from gestation to adolescence. Prev Chronic Dis 2009;6(3). http://www.cdc.gov/pcd/issues jul/09_0014.htm. Accessed [01/26/ 2009].
[38] Berenson, GS; Srinivasan, SR; Bao, W; Newman, WP; 3rd; Tracy, RE; Wattigney, WA. Association between multiple cardiovascular risk factors and atherosclerosis in children and young adults. The Bogalusa Heart Study. *N Engl J Med.*, 1998, Jun 4,

338(23), 1650-6.

[39] Center for Disease Control. Diabetes Data & Trends. Number (in Millions) of Civilian/Noninstitutionalized Persons with Diagnosed Diabetes, United States, 1980–2006. Available at http://www.cdc.gov/diabetes ational/figpersons.htm. *Accessed January*, 19, 2010.

[40] Centers for Disease Control and Prevention. National diabetes fact sheet: general information and national estimates on diabetes in the United States, 2007. Atlanta, GA: U.S. Department of Health and Human Services, Centers for Disease Control and Prevention, 2008.

[41] Visscher, TL; Seidell, JC. The public health impact of obesity. *Annu Rev Public Health,* 2001, 22, 355-75.

[42] Liese, AD; D'Agostino, RB; Jr., Hamman, RF; Kilgo, PD; Lawrence, JM; Liu, LL; et al. The burden of diabetes mellitus among US youth: prevalence estimates from the SEARCH for Diabetes in Youth Study. *Pediatrics*, 2006, Oct;118(4), 1510-8.

[43] Bell, RA; Mayer-Davis, EJ; Beyer, JW; D'Agostino, RB; Jr., Lawrence, JM; Linder, B; et al. Diabetes in non-Hispanic white youth: prevalence, incidence, and clinical characteristics: the SEARCH for Diabetes in Youth Study. *Diabetes Care*, 2009, Mar;32 Suppl 2, S102-S111.

[44] Bell, RA; Mayer-Davis, EJ; Beyer, JW; D'Agostino, RB; Jr., Lawrence, JM; Linder, B; et al. Diabetes in non-Hispanic white youth: prevalence, incidence, and clinical characteristics: the SEARCH for Diabetes in Youth Study. *Diabetes Care*, 2009, Mar, 32 Suppl 2, S102-S111.

[45] Petitti, DB; Klingensmith, GJ; Bell, RA; Andrews, JS; Dabelea, D; Imperatore, G; et al. Glycemic control in youth with diabetes: the SEARCH for diabetes in Youth Study. *J Pediatr*, 2009, Nov;155(5), 668-72.

[46] Arenz, S; Ruckerl, R; Koletzko, B; et al. Breast- feeding and childhood obesity—a systematic review. [Review] Int J Obes Relat Metab Disord: Journal of the International Association for the *Study of Obesity*, 2004, 28, 1247-1256.

[47] Division of Nutrition and Physical Activity. Research to Practices Series No. 3: Does Drinking Beverages with Added Sugars Increase the Risk of Overweight? Atlanta: *Centers for Disease Control and Prevention*, 2006.

[48] Coon, KA; Tucker, KL. Television and children's consumption patterns. A review of the literature. *Minerva Pediatr*, 2002, 54, 423-436.

[49] Björntorp, P. Do stress reactions cause abdominal obesity and comorbidities? *Obes Rev,* 2001, 2(2), 73-86.

[50] Braveman, P. A health disparities perspective on obesity research. *Prev Chronic Dis*, 2009, 6(3).

[51] U.S. Department of Health and Human Services. U.S. Department of Agriculture. Dietary Guidelines for Americans, 2005, 6th edition, Washington, D.C.: U.S. Government Printing Office, January 2005.

[52] Dennison, BA; Television Viewing and Television in Bedrooms Associated with Overweight Risk Among Low-Income Preschool Children, Pediatrics, 2002, 109(9), 1028-1035.

[53] 2008 Physical Activity Guidelines for Americans. Available at http://www.health. Accessed December 31, 2009.

[54] Rideout, V; Vanderwater, E; Wartella, E. Kaiser Family Foundation; Generation M2:

Media in the Lives of 8- to 18-Year-Olds, January 20, 2010.
[55] Kaiser Family Foundation. Zero to six: electronic media in the lives of infants, toddlers and preschoolers. Menlo Park (CA): The Henry *J. Kaiser Family Foundation*; 2003.
[56] Forum on Child and Family Statistics. America's Children: Key National Indicators of Well-Being 2009. Available at http://www.childstats.gov/americaschildren/f amsoc3.asp. *Accessed December*, 29, 2009.
[57] Centers for Disease Control and Prevention. Guidelines for school and community programs to promote lifelong physical activity among young people. MMWR. 1997, 46 (No. RR-6):1-36
[58] Centers for Disease Control and Prevention. Guidelines for school health programs to promote lifelong healthy eating. MMWR. 1996, 45(No. RR-9):1-41
[59] Gortmaker, SL; Peterson, K; Wiecha, J; Sobol, AM; Dixit, S; Fox, MK; Laird, N. Reducing obesity via a school-based interdisciplinary intervention among youth: Planet Health. *Arch Pediatr Adolesc Med.*, 1999, 53(4), 409- 418.
[60] Robinson, TN. Reducing children's television viewing to prevent obesity: a randomized controlled trial. *JAMA.*, 1999, 282(16), 1561-1567.
[61] Coleman, KJ; Tiller, CL; Sanchez, J; Heath, EM; Sy, O; Milliken, G; Dzewaltowski, DA. Prevention of the epidemic increase in child risk of overweight in low-income schools: The El Paso Coordinated Approach to Child Health. *Arch Pediatr Adolesc Med.*, 2005, 159(3), 21 7-224.
[62] Economos, CD; Hyatt, RR; Goldberg, JP; Must, A; Naumova, EN; Collins, JJ; Nelson, ME. A community intervention reduces BMI z-score in children: Shape Up Somerville first year results. *Obesity.*, 2007, 5(5), 1325-1336.
[63] Foster, GD; Sherman, S; Borradaile, KE; Grundy, KM; Vander Veur, SS; Nachmani, J; Karpyn, A; Kumanyika, S; Shultz, J. A policy- based school intervention to prevent overweight and obesity. *Pediatrics.*, 2008, 121(4), e794-e802.
[64] Gutin, B; Yin, Z; Johnson, M; Barbeau, P. Preliminary findings of the effect of a 3-year after-school physical activity intervention on fitness and body fat: The Medical College of Georgia Fitkid Project. *Int J Pediatr Obes.*, 2008, 3(Suppl 1):3-9.
[65] National Association for Sport and Physical Education. Understanding the difference: is it physical education or physical activity? Reston (VA): National Association for Sport and Physical Education; 2005. Available at http://www.aahperd.org/naspe/publications/ te achingTools/PAvsPE.cfm. Accessed on December 31, 2009.
[66] National Association for Sport and Physical Education. Comprehensive school physical activity programs. Reston (VA): National Association for Sport and Physical Education; 2008. Available at http://www.aahperd.org/naspe/standards/uplo ad/Comprehensive-School-Physical-ActivityPrograms-2008.pdf. Accessed on December 31, 2009.
[67] Lee, SM; Burgeson, CR; Fulton, JE; Spain, CC. Physical education and physical activity: results from the School Health Policies and Programs Study, 2006, *J Sch Health.* 2007, 77(8), 435-463.
[68] Centers for Disease Control and Prevention. Youth Risk Behavior Surveillance — United States, 2007. Surveillance Summaries, 2008. *MMWR.* 2008;57(No. SS–4):1-131.
[69] Anderson, LM; Quinn, TA; Glanz, K; Ramirez, G; Kahwati, LC; Johnson, DB; Buchanan, LR; Archer, WR; Chattopadhyay, S; Kalra, GP; Katz, DL; Task Force on

Community Preventive Services. The effectiveness of worksite nutrition and physical activity interventions for controlling employee overweight and obesity: a systematic review. *Am J Prev Med.*, 2009, Oct;37(4), 340-57. Review.

[70] Finkelstein, EA; Trogdon, JG; Cohen, JW; Dietz, W. Annual medical spending attributable to obesity: payer-and service- specific estimates. Health Affairs (Millwood). 2009, Sep-Oct;28(5), w822-31. *Epub*, 2009, Jul 27.

[71] Thorpe, KE; Florence, CS; Howard, DH; Joski, P. The impact of obesity on rising medical ppending. *Health Affairs (Millwood),* 2004, W4, 480-486.

[72] Aldana, SG. Financial Impact of Health Promotion Programs: A comprehensive review of the literature. *Am J Health Promot.*, 2001, 15(5), 296-320.

[73] Chapman, LS. Meta-evaluation of worksite health promotion economic return studies: 2005 Update. *Am J Health Promot.*, 2005, 19(6), 1-11.

[74] Goetzel, RZ; Ozminkowski, RJ. The health and cost benefits of work site health-promotion programs. *Annu Rev Public Health*, 2008, 29, 303-323.

[75] Pelletier, KR. A review and analysis of the clinical and cost-effectiveness studies of comprehensive health promotion and disease management programs at the worksite: 2000-2004 update (VI). *J Occup Environ Med.*, 2005, 47(10), 1051-1058.

[76] Center for Disease Control. CDC's LEAN Works! – A workplace obesity prevention program. Available at http://www.cdc.gov/LEANWorks/. Accessed on December, 31, 2009.

[77] Phillips, RL; Jr; Bazemore, AW; Dodoo, MS; Shipman, SA; Green, LA. Family physicians in the child health care workforce: opportunities for collaboration in improving the health of children. *Pediatrics*, 2006, 188(3), 1200-6.

[78] Whitlock, EP; O'Connor, EA; Williams, SB; Beil, TL; Lutz, KW. Effectiveness of weight management interventions in children: A targeted systematic review for the USPSTF. *Pediatrics*, 2010, 10. 1542/peds.2009-1955.

[79] Khan, L; Sobush, K; Keener, D; Goodman, K; Lowry, A; Kakietek, J; Zaro, S. Recommended community strategies and measurements to prevent obesity in the United States. *MMWR*, 58, RR-7, 2009.

In: Solving Childhood Obesity
Editors: Sarah J. Maier and Natalie E. Brunner

ISBN: 978-1-61209-964-4

Chapter 4

OBESITY PREVALENCE AMONG LOW-INCOME, PRESCHOOL-AGED CHILDREN —UNITED STATES, 1998–2008

Centers for Disease Control and Prevention

Childhood obesity continues to be a leading public health concern that disproportionately affects low-income and minority children [1]. Children who are obese in their preschool years are more likely to be obese in adolescence and adulthood [2] and to develop diabetes, hypertension, hyperlipidemia, asthma, and sleep apnea [3]. One of the *Healthy People 2010* objectives (19-3) is to reduce to 5% the proportion of children and adolescents who are obese [4]. CD C's Pediatric Nutrition Surveillance System (PedNSS) is the only source of nationally compiled obesity surveillance data obtained at the state and local level for low-income, preschool-aged children participating in federally funded health and nutrition programs. To describe progress in reducing childhood obesity, CDC examined trends and current prevalence in obesity using PedNSS data submitted by participating states, territories, and Indian tribal organizations during 1998–2008. The findings indicated that obesity prevalence among low-income, preschool-aged children increased steadily from 12.4% in 1998 to 14.5% in 2003, but subsequently remained essentially the same, with a 14.6% prevalence in 2008. Reducing childhood obesity will require effective prevention strategies that focus on environments and policies promoting physical activity and a healthy diet for families, child care centers, and communities.

PedNSS is a state-based surveillance system that monitors the nutritional status of children from birth through age 4 years enrolled in federally funded programs that serve low-income children. For all states except California and North Carolina, data come exclusively from the Special Supplemental Nutrition Program for Women, Infants, and Children (WIC).*

* Eligibility criteria for WIC includes a family income ≤185% of the poverty income threshold, based on U.S. Poverty Income Guidelines, available at http:// aspe.os.dhhs.gov/poverty. A person who participates or has family members who participate in certain other benefit programs, such as the Medicaid or Aid to Families with Dependent Children/Temporary Assistance to Needy Families, automatically meets the income-eligibility requirement.

In California, data are exclusively from Medicaid-funded programs. North Carolina submits data from both WIC (95.5%) and non-WIC programs (4.5%).[†] For the states included in this analysis, 21.0% of children aged 2–4 years are covered by PedNSS. On average, children are seen twice a year by the program; height and weight are measured each time. Data are collected at the clinic level and submitted to CDC for analysis. Federally funded programs submit data on weight, height (measured by trained staff using a standard protocol during clinic visits), age, sex, and the race/ethnicity reported by the child's parent or caregiver. CDC uses weight, height, and age data to calculate body mass index (BMI) (weight [kg] / height [m^2]). For children aged 2–4 years, obesity is defined as BMIfor-age >95th percentile based on the 2000 CDC sex-specific growth charts[5]. CDC performs routine edits to assess data quality. An error flag is applied to height or weight data that are either missing, miscoded, or biologically implausible (e.g., height-for-age z-score <-5.0 or >3.0, body mass index [BMI]- for-age [children aged ≥2 years] z-score <-4.0 or >5.0, weightfor-age z-score <-4.0 or >5.0, or BMI-for-age [children aged ≥2 years] z-score <-4.0 or >5.0). All flagged data are excluded from PedNSS analyses.

The *MMWR* series of publications is published by the Coordinating Center for Health Information and Service, Centers for Disease Control and Prevention (CDC), U.S. Department of Health and Human Services, Atlanta, GA 30333.

Suggested Citation: Centers for Disease Control and Prevention. [Article title]. MMWR 2009;58: [inclusive page numbers].

[†] Including the Early and Periodic Screening, Diagnosis, and Treatment Program, other Medicaid-funded child health programs, and Title V Maternal and Child Health Programs. Eligibility criteria includes a family income <200% of the poverty income threshold, based on U.S. Poverty Income Guidelines. The non- WIC records accounted for 24% of records in 1998, 19% in 2003, and 15% in 2008.

CDC randomly selected one record per child per year to estimate obesity prevalence in 1998, 2003, and 2008. To assess the change in obesity prevalence in PedNSS overall and by race/ethnicity, prevalence was estimated using data only from the subset of federally funded programs that participated in 1998, 2003, and 2008 (N = 37). The average annual change in obesity prevalence during 1998–2003 and 2003–2008 was estimated for each PedNSS program. If data for a program were unavailable for a given year but were available for the preceding or subsequent year, CDC substituted the data for the adjacent year and calculated the annual change to account for the shorter or longer period. Chi-square tests for difference in proportions were conducted across each period, and tests were statistically significant ($p<0.05$) unless otherwise noted in this report.

During 1998–2008, the number of federally funded programs reporting data to PedNSS varied from 43 to 52. In 2008, records on approximately 8 million children were submitted from 43 states, the District of Columbia, Puerto Rico, the U.S. Virgin Islands, and six Indian tribal organizations (Table). The overall prevalence of obesity among low-income, preschool-aged children increased from 12.4% (n = 1,999,970) in 1998 to 14.5% (n = 1,967,625) in 2003 and 14.6% (n = 2,222,410) in 2008 (Figure). Obesity prevalence increased 0.43 percentage points annually during 1998–2003, but only 0.02 percentage points annually during 2003–2008. Obesity increased across all racial/ethnic groups during 1998–2003, with the exception of Asian/Pacific Islander (A/PI) children. However, during 2003–2008, obesity remained stable among all groups except American Indian/Alaska Native (AI/AN) children. In 2008, prevalence was highest among AI/AN (21.2%) and Hispanic (18.5%) children, and lowest among non-Hispanic white (12.6%), non-Hispanic black (11.8%), and A/PI (12.3%) children.

In 2008, only programs in Colorado and Hawaii had obesity prevalences ≤10%. The two federally funded programs with prevalence >20% were Indian tribal organizations (Table). Of the 41 PedNSS programs supplying data for 1998–2003, a total of 38 (93%) reported an increase in obesity prevalence. In contrast, of the 44 programs supplying data for 2003–2008, 22 (50%) reported an increase in obesity, whereas 14 (32%) reported no change, and eight (18%) reported a decrease.

Reported by: *AJ Sharma, PhD, LM Grummer-Strawn, PhD, K Dalenius, MPH, D Galuska, PhD, M Anandappa, MS, E Borland, H Mackintosh, MSPH, R Smith, MS, Div of Nutrition, Physical Activity and Obesity, National Center for Chronic Disease Prevention and Health Promotion, CDC.*

Editorial Note: Reduction of obesity among children and adolescents is a national priority in the United States [4]. The results presented in this report indicate that among low-income, preschool-aged children participating in federally funded nutrition programs, the prevalence of obesity increased during 1998–2003, but stabilized during 2003–2008. In 2008, the national prevalence of obesity in this group remained highest among low-income Hispanic and AI/AN children and continued to increase among AI/AN children. These results suggest overall progress in stabilizing the prevalence of childhood obesity in a subset of low-income, preschool-aged children. However, these results should be confirmed through additional research using other data sets.

Table. 1 Average annual change in obesity* prevalence among children aged 2–4 years, by state, territory, and Indian tribal organization† — Pediatric Nutrition Surveillance System, United States, 1998–2003 and 2003–2008.

State, territory, or Indian tribal organization	1998		2003		2008		Average percentage-point change per year	
	No. of children	Obesity prevalence (%)	No. of children	Obesity prevalence (%)	No. of children	Obesity prevalence (%)	1998–2003	2003–2008
Alabama	39,998	11.7	30,221	14.7†	56,813	13.8	0.59	-0.23
Arizona	51,279	9.7	67,618	12.4†	75,338	14.6	0.45	0.55
Arkansas	34,968	9.7	31,625	12.2	38,591	13.9	0.50	0.34
California	398,222	15.5	344,384	17.6	301,643	17.3	0.42	-0.06
Colorado	— §	—	50,773	9.4	43,476	9.4	—	0.00**
Connecticut	23,272	17.8	22,495	19.6	25,623	15.5	0.36	-0.82
Florida	141,831	11.3	155,482	13.4	209,671	14.1	0.42	0.14
Georgia	87,823	9.4	92,728	12.4	124,533	14.8	0.60	0.48
Hawaii	3,649	10.3	15,602	10.1	16,106	9.3	-0.04**	-0.16
Idaho	15,121	9.8	16,340	11.2	20,081	12.3	0.28	0.22
Illinois	88,178	13.5	70,666	13.9	63,414	14.7	0.08	0.16
Indiana	64,411	10.5	51,953	13.7	66,499	14.5	0.64	0.16
Iowa	29,788	10.6	32,913	13.9	33,548	15.1	0.66	0.24
Kansas	22,628	8.8	27,076	12.6	34,352	13.3	0.76	0.14
Kentucky	48,075	12.1	60,984	17.2	62,832	15.7	1.02	-0.30
Louisiana	45,834	10.4	44,036	13.3	34,041	13.8¶	0.58	0.13
Maine	11,747	12.1	9,861	15.8	—	—	0.74	—
Maryland	23,329	12.0	42,884	14.4†	54,866	15.7	0.40	0.33
Massachusetts	59,511	14.8	55,785	16.7	59,297	16.7	0.38	0.00**
Michigan	90,760	10.1	93,962	12.9	103,523	13.9	0.56	0.20
Minnesota	76,271	11.0	40,161	13.2	65,607	13.4	0.44	0.04**
Mississippi	11,850	13.2	—	—	44,807	14.6	—	—
Missouri	58,000	9.8	56,346	13.3	60,908	13.9	0.70	0.12

Table 1 (Continued).

State, territory, or Indian tribal organization	1998		2003		2008		Average percentage-point change per year	
	No. of children	Obesity prevalence (%)	No. of children	Obesity prevalence (%)	No. of children	Obesity prevalence (%)	1998–2003	2003–2008
Montana	9,658	9.0	10,178	11.0	10,428	12.4	0.40	0.28
Nebraska	13,961	9.9	17,242	13.4	20,658	13.9	0.70	0.10**
Nevada	6,123	11.6	14,595	13.6	23,348	12.9	0.40	-0.14
New Hampshire	5,530	13.5	7,227	15.6	8,082	15.5	0.42	-0.02**
New Jersey	56,292	15.1	56,774	17.9	68,163	17.9	0.56	0.00**
New Mexico	17,523	7.6	27,555	9.7	22,295	12.0	0.42	0.46
New York	207,479	14.7	186,284	16.6	209,713	14.6	0.38	-0.40
North Carolina	80,956	11.1	75,206	14.5	96,381	15.7	0.68	0.24
North Dakota	7,246	9.4	6,097	11.6	6,551	13.8	0.44	0.44
Ohio	17,219	10.4	89,824	11.6	125,011	12.2	0.24	0.12
Oregon	34,546	11.9	29,875	14.7	49,193	14.7	0.56	0.00**
Pennsylvania	108,858	10.7	100,053	12.4	111,879	11.5	0.34	-0.18
Rhode Island	—	—	—	—	11,466	16.2	—	—
South Carolina	48,543	10.0	32,239	12.4	28,209	13.3	0.48	0.18
South Dakota	8,968	9.0	8,423	13.6	9,125	16.2	0.92	0.52
Tennessee	56,208	10.0	60,086	12.0	49,016	13.8	0.40	0.36
Texas	—	—	422,127	14.4	164,435	16.2	—	0.36
Utah	23,765	6.5	31,099	8.6	—	—	0.42	—
Vermont	6,225	11.6	8,504	13.1	7,009	13.3	0.30	0.04**
Virginia	—	—	20,238	18.5	59,627	19.0	—	0.10**
Washington	55,162	12.0	65,828	13.8¶	92,980	14.4	0.45	0.10
West Virginia	24,170	10.6	22,079	13.2	22,689	13.5	0.52	0.06**
Wisconsin	52,186	10.1	50,284	13.0	55,875	13.6	0.58	0.12
Wyoming	—	—	5,269	9.5	—	—	—	—

State, territory, or Indian tribal organization	1998		2003		2008		Average percentage-point change per year	
	No. of children	Obesity prevalence (%)	No. of children	Obesity prevalence (%)	No. of children	Obesity prevalence (%)	1998–2003	2003–2008
District of Columbia	6,499	10.9	5,926	13.3	6,195	13.3	0.48	0.00**
Puerto Rico	—	—	102,624	24.0	99,829	17.9	—	-1.22
U.S. Virgin Islands	—	—	—	—	2,339	13.6	—	—
Cheyenne River Sioux Tribe (SD)	362	22.1†	388	17.5	423	18.4	-1.15**	0.18**
Chickasaw Nation (OK)	1,039	8.9	1,478	12.0	—	—	0.62	—
Inter Tribal Council of Arizona	4,680	19.8	5,037	20.9	5,823	23.5	0.22**	0.52
Navajo Nation	—	—	7,616	14.4	6,824	16.9	—	0.50
Rosebud Sioux Tribe (SD)	604	16.4	641	17.3	651	19.2	0.18**	0.38**
Standing Rock Sioux Tribe (ND)	—	—	422	20.1	541	25.0	—	0.98**
Three Affiliated Tribes (ND)	—	—	—	—	163	19.6	—	—

* Defined as body mass index (BMI)-for-age >95th percentile based on the 2000 CDC sex-specific growth charts, available at http://www.cdc.gov/growthcharts.
† Data from subsequent year used.
§ Data not available.
¶ Data from preceding year used.
** No significant change in obesity prevalence.

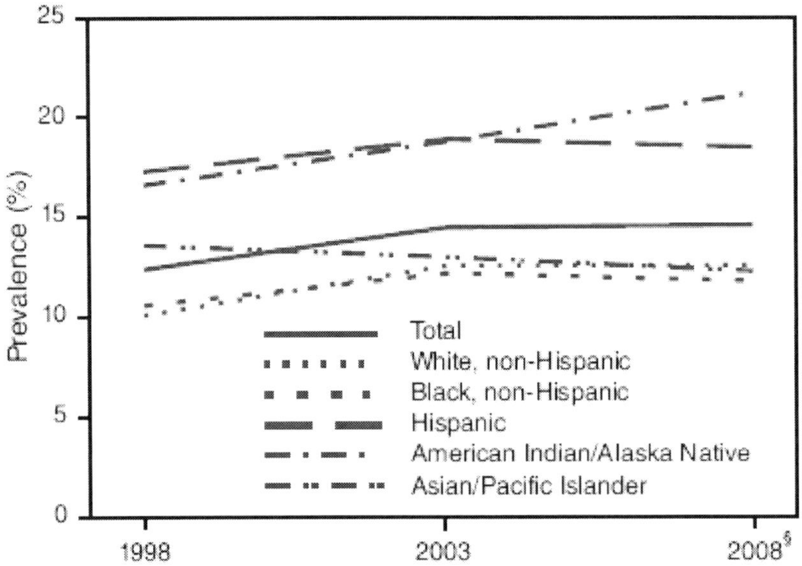

* Defined as body mass index (BMI)-for-age >95th percentile based on the 2000 CDC sex-specific growth charts, available at http://www.cdc.gov/growth charts.

† Includes only the 37 federally funded programs that provided data in 1998, 2003, and 2008.

§ Sample sizes in 2008 were as follows: total, 2,222,410; non-Hispanic white, 845,910; non-Hispanic black, 438,645; Hispanic, 749,1 09; American Indian/Alaska Native, 23,960; and Asian/Pacific Islander, 68,933.

Figure1. Change in obesity* prevalence during 1998–2003 and 2003–2008 among children aged 2–4 years, by race/ ethnicity — Pediatric Nutrition Surveillance System, United States, 1998–2008†.

Children in preschool age groups are a priority for surveillance because obesity trends in this group can serve as a bellwether for trends in older children and adults (*2*). PedNSS currently serves as the only source of national obesity prevalence data compiled specifically on low-income, preschool-aged children. Because PedNSS nutritional data are dependent on enrollments in participating federally funded programs, PedNSS results are subject to variations in enrollment in these programs in each state. However, the effect of such variations on PedNSS results is difficult to determine. Conditions within a state that differentially affect the enrollment of children with varying prevalences of obesity could affect state or national results. In addition, changes in the proportion of children from each state might alter the results. For example, California, the largest data contributor to PedNSS, has one of the highest prevalences of obesity. The percentage of the total PedNSS sample provided by California decreased from 20.2% in 1998 to 13.6% in 2008. However, even deletion of all California data would not alter the overall results; an increase from 1998 to 2003 would still be observed, followed by stabilization through 2008. Furthermore, stabilization or declines were observed in half of the individual federally funded programs in PedNSS.

To maintain the consistency of PedNSS data, methods for data collection and recording are set nationally and are uniform across states and participating federal programs. The procedures for collecting height and weight data did not change during 1998–2008, with the exception of an increasing use of digital scales. Given the procedures within the WIC program for regular calibration of scales, this change should not affect rates of obesity. CDC has stringent requirements for data quality and uses standardized procedures for data cleaning; data files that do not meet these standards are rejected, as are records that do not meet standards for acceptable heights and weights.

The reason for the stabilization of overall obesity prevalence among these children during 2003–2008 is not known and likely is complex. One factor might be prevention efforts within state and local WIC programs targeting behaviors related to obesity in children. For example, certain initiatives in WIC[§] have attempted to raise public awareness, acceptance, and support of breastfeeding, increased the percentage of low-fat or fat-free milk vouchers issued for children aged >2 years,[¶] and reduced television viewing [6]. Recommendations such as those from the Institute of Medicine's *Preventing Childhood Obesity* report also might have spurred greater attention to obesity prevention for all children [7].

The National Health and Nutrition Examination Survey (NHANES) also has found a stabilization of obesity prevalence in U.S. children. NHANES found no significant increase in obesity prevalence during 1999–2006 in children aged 2–19 years [8]. This apparent plateau remained even after adjusting for differences in prevalence by age group. Trends in the 2–5 year age group were not analyzed separately because of small sample size. For NHANES 2003–2006, the overall prevalence of obesity (BMI-for-age ≥ 95th percentile) for children aged 2–5 years was 12.4% (standard error = 1.0%), lower than the rates for both 2003 and 2008 described in this report.

The findings in this report are subject to at least three limitations. First, the proportion of children participating in federally funded nutrition programs increased during 1998–2008, as evidenced by the 11% increase in the number of children in these analyses (i.e., from 1,999,970 in 1998 to 2,222,410 in 2008). However, how the addition of these children might have affected the prevalence of obesity is unknown. Second, the percentage of the total PedNSS dataset that is made up of WIC records increased from 76% in 1998 to 85% in 2008. If the prevalence of obesity were lower in WIC than in non-WIC programs, this increase could partially explain the observed trends. However, when the analysis was conducted using only data from WIC, results were not substantially different. Finally, PedNSS data are not representative of all low-income, preschool-aged children in the United States because not all states participate in PedNSS and not all low-income children participate in federally funded programs.

Childhood obesity remains a serious public health problem even among this subset, particularly among AI/AN children. A sustained and effective public health response is necessary across the United States to reduce childhood obesity. Strategies should emphasize improving environments and policies that promote physical activity and a healthy diet.

References

[1] Wang, Y; Beydoun, MA. The obesity epidemic in the United States—gender, age, socioeconomic, racial/ethnic, and geographic characteristics: a systematic review and

[§] Additional information available at http://www.nal.usda.gov/wicworks/ spotlight/bfweek_resources.html.
Additional information available at http://www.health nutrition/resources/docs/2003-2006_ewph_community_intervention_projects. pdf.

meta-regression analysis. *Epidemiol Rev*, 2007, 29, 6–28.

[2] Serdula, MK; Ivery, D; Coates, RJ; Freedman, DS; Williamson, DF; Byers, T. Do obese children become obese adults? A review of the literature. *Prev Med*, 1993, 22, 167–77.

[3] American Academy of Pediatrics. Policy statement: prevention of pediatric overweight and obesity. *Pediatrics*, 2003, 112, 424–30.

[4] US Department of Health and Human Services. Healthy people 2010: objectives for improving health (part B: focus areas 15–28). 2nd ed. Washington, DC: US Department of Health and Human Services; 2000. Available at http://www. health.gov/healthypeople.

[5] Kuczmarski, RJ; Ogden, CL; Grummer-Strawn, LM; et al. CDC growth charts: United States. Adv Data 2000;314: 1–27. Available at http://www. cdc.gov/growthcharts.

[6] Johnson, DB; Birkett, D; Evens, C; Pickering, S. Statewide intervention to reduce television viewing in WIC clients and staff. *Am J Health Promot,* 2005, 19, 418–21.

[7] Institute of Medicine. Preventing childhood obesity: health in the balance. Washington, DC: National Academies Press; 2005.

[8] Ogden, CL; Carroll, MD; Flegal, KM. High body mass index for age among US children and adolescents, 2003–2006. *JAMA*, 2008, 299, 2401–5.

Neurologic Complications Associated with Novel Influenza A (H1N 1) Virus Infection in Children —Dallas, Texas, May 2009

Neurologic complications, including seizures, encephalitis, encephalopathy, Reye syndrome, and other neurologic disorders, have been described previously in association with respiratory tract infection with seasonal influenza A or B viruses [1–2], but not with novel influenza A (H1N1) virus. On May 28, 2009, the Dallas County Department of Health and Human Services (DCHHS) notified CDC of four children with neurologic complications associated with novel influenza A (H1N1) virus infection admitted to hospitals in Dallas County, Texas, during May 18–28. This report summarizes the clinical characteristics of those four cases. Patients were aged 7–17 years and were admitted with signs of influenza-like illness (ILI) and seizures or altered mental status. Three of the four patients had abnormal electroencephalograms (EEGs). In all four patients, novel influenza A (H 1N 1) viral RNA was detected in nasopharyngeal specimens but not in cerebrospinal fluid (CSF). Antiviral therapy included oseltamivir (four patients) and rimantadine (three patients). All four patients recovered fully and had no neurologic sequelae at discharge. These findings indicate that, as with seasonal influenza, neurologic complications can occur after respiratory tract infection with novel influenza A (H1N1) virus. For children who have ILI accompanied by unexplained seizures or mental status changes, clinicians should consider acute seasonal influenza or novel influenza A (H 1N 1) virus infection in the differential diagnosis, send respiratory specimens for appropriate diagnostic testing, and promptly initiate empirical antiviral treatment, especially in hospitalized patients.

Case Identification

Since April 22, DCHHS has requested all hospitals in Dallas County to report details concerning patients admitted with novel influenza A (H1N1) virus infection. As of July 20, DCHHS had identified 405 persons with laboratory-confirmed novel influenza A (H1N1) virus infection in the greater Dallas area, including 44 hospitalized patients. No deaths had been reported. Of confirmed novel influenza A (H1N1) virus infections, 83% were in patients aged <18 years. Among these pediatric cases, 145 children, including 26 who were hospitalized, were identified through the Children's Medical Center of Dallas (CMCD) laboratory- based surveillance program. Medical records from admission and discharge for all hospitalized H 1N 1 patients are routinely

In: Solving Childhood Obesity
Editors: Sarah J. Maier and Natalie E. Brunner
ISBN: 978-1-61209-964-4

Chapter 5

REDUCING CHILDREN'S TV TIME TO REDUCE THE RISK OF CHILDHOOD OVERWEIGHT: THE CHILDREN'S MEDIA USE STUDY

Centers for Disease Control and Prevention

ACKNOWLEDGMENTS

This study was conceived and funded by the Nutrition and Physical Activity Communication team in CDC's Division of Nutrition and Physical Activity. The study was conducted by RTI International, James Hersey, Ph.D., Principal Investigator (P.I.), and the Annenberg Public Policy Center of the University of Pennsylvania, Amy Jordan, Ph.D., Co-P.I., under a cooperative agreement with the Association for Prevention Teaching and Research (Cooperative Agreement No. TS-8046). The Technical Advisor for this study was Judith McDivitt, Ph.D.

Members of the study team are listed below.

Children's Media Use Study Team

RTI	APPC	CDC Consultants
James Hersey, Ph.D., P.I. Lucia Rojas Smith, Ph.D. Holly Massett, Ph.D. Rosanna Quiros, Ph.D. Jeanette Renaud, Ph.D. Christina An Finkelstein, M.A. Sally Salib, B.A. Peyton Williams, B.A.	Amy Jordan, Ph.D., Co-P.I. Amy Branner, Ph.D. Jennifer Horner, Ph.D. Sharon Tellen, Ph.D., University of Illinois at Chicago	Judith McDivitt, Ph.D. Carrie Heitzler, M.P.H. Arlynn Filomeno, M.P.H. Janet Fulton, Ph.D. Larry Grummer-Straum, Ph.D.

1. Study Background, Objectives, and Approach

1.1. Study Background

Although there is a long history of public concern over the impact of mass media on children's psychosocial development (Center on Media and Child Health 2005; Lowery and DeFleur 1995), it is only in the past two decades that researchers have begun to uncover the link between media use and the physical health of youths. Data from large-scale national surveys conducted during the 1980s and 1990s reveal a correlation between the prevalence of overweight and the number of hours youths spend watching TV (Andersen et al. 1998; Dietz and Gortmaker 1985). More importantly, subsequent longitudinal studies (Gortmaker et al. 1996) and field experiments (Robinson1999) have indicated a potential causal connection between obesity/overweight and heavy TV use.

The parallel increase in the amount of media available to children and the prevalence of overweight in America's children is probably not coincidental. A national survey by the Annenberg Public Policy Center (APPC) (based on 1,235 parents of 2- to 17-year-olds and 416 children and adolescents aged 8- to 16.) indicates that today's homes are saturated with media (Woodard and Gridina, 2000). The majority of the families in these studies have three TVs, access to cable or satellite channels, at least one VCR, a videogame system, and a computer with online access. Children's bedrooms themselves have become multimedia centers: more than half (57 %) of 8- to 16-year-olds have a TV in their bedroom; 39 % have videogame equipment; 30 % have a VCR; 20 % have a computer; and 11 % have access to the Internet.

Although 39 percent of parents in the APPC national survey said that they have limits for how much time their child can spend watching TV, significantly more said they had rules about completing chores or homework before watching (68 %) and the kinds of programs their child can watch (50 %). Indeed, parents are much more likely to say that they are concerned about what their child watches on TV (64 %) than they are to express concern over how much time their child spends watching TV (21 %).

It is perhaps not surprising—given easy access and a general lack of parental concern about the amount of TV use—that the average child on an average day will spend 4.5 hours looking at a screen of some type (APPC 2000). Although the amount of time children spend watching TV has remained fairly constant over the past decade, children have supplemented this time with additional sedentary media activity, including time spent online and engaged in videogame play.

Similarly, a 2003 national survey of children, sponsored by the Kaiser Family Foundation, indicates that the average child between the ages of 8 and 18 watches 3 hours of TV a day, and the averages are even higher among younger age groups (8- to 14-year-olds watched an average of 3 hours and 16 minutes). Total in-home screen time rises to 4 hours and 15 minutes when videos and DVDs are included. The addition of computers and videogames raises total exposure to more than 6 hours (Roberts, Foehr, and Rideout 2005).

Gortmaker et al. (1996) point out that the factors associated with the substantial hours of TV viewing are not well understood, and, in their analysis of a nationally representative sample of 6- to 11-year-olds with a 4-year follow-up, they write that "very little predicts TV viewing in this sample" (p. 360). Other studies, however, have linked high levels of media use to low socioeconomic status, heavy parental media use, and ethnic minority status (Gorley, Marshall, and Biddle 2004; Roberts et al. 1999; Woodard and Gridina 2000).

At the same time that media have proliferated in children's lives, public health experts and organizations, including the Centers for Disease Control and Prevention (CDC), have raised alarms over the steady increase in the prevalence of child overweight and obesity (Institute of Medicine 2005). Results from the 1999 to 2002 National Health and Nutrition Examination Survey (NHANES) indicate that 16 percent of children and adolescents aged 6 to 19 years are overweight. This figure represents a 45 percent increase from the overweight estimates of 11 percent obtained from NHANES III (1988 to 1994) (Hedley et al. 2004). Being overweight during childhood has been shown to be more than a cosmetic issue. Mossberg (1989), for example, followed 500 overweight children over the course of 40 years at 10-year intervals and found that, in addition to obesity in the family, the degree of overweight in puberty was the most important predictor of adulthood body weight. These studies found an association between overweight in childhood and adult morbidity and mortality.

The problem of obesity has hit children in racial and ethnic minority groups especially hard. Strauss and Pollack (2001), examining data from the National Longitudinal Survey of Youth (1986 to 1998), found that the prevalence of overweight increased fastest among these groups. By 1998, 21.5 percent of African American, 21.8 percent of nonwhite Hispanic, and 12.3 percent of white children were deemed to be overweight. Adolescent females, perhaps because they are less likely to participate in sports teams or physical play, are also at greater risk for overweight than are adolescent males and appear to be more negatively affected by heavy TV use (Anderson et al. 1998).

The association between TV use and overweight in children may result from (1) displacement of more active pursuits and/or decreased energy expenditure and (2) increased caloric intake resulting from greater snacking opportunities and poorer food choices. Several authors, including Crespo et al. (2001), Gortmaker et al. (1996), and Robinson (1999) posit that TV use may displace physical activity but also increase caloric intake during viewing and increase interest in purchasing the high-fat, high-sugar, nutritionally empty products children see advertised. Surveys that track children's eating habits and nutritional choices suggest that TV influences both how much and what children eat (Crespo et al. 2001; Signorelli and Staples 1997). More research is needed to explain the causal mechanism between TV use and overweight. Moreover, we do not know the extent to which use of non-TV media, such as videogames, might have similar consequences. For example, Signorelli and Staples (1997) argue that children not only are sedentary while viewing but are tempted to overeat because they see food advertisements and have free hands to engage in snacking behaviors.

Nonetheless, there is mounting experimental evidence that reducing TV use can have a positive impact on children's weight. Researchers at Stanford University designed an intervention that targeted media use alone, without substituting alternative behaviors such as physical activity. In the intervention schools, third- and fourth-graders were exposed to a media literacy curriculum that emphasized choice of TV programs to watch, and were encouraged to limit their TV, videotape, and videogame use. The children in this intervention group had statistically significant relative decreases in body mass index (BMI) when compared with matched children in a control condition (Robinson, 1999). Similarly, Robinson et al. (2003) found that, among low-income 8–10 year old African American girls, an after-school dance class coupled with family intervention to reduce TV use, resulted in a lowering of BMI among the intervention group compared with a control group. A study in Massachusetts of a school-based intervention with children aged 6-8 that included a TV reduction component found a significant reduction in obesity among girls, though not among boys, and found that this reduction was mediated by changes in TV viewing (Gortmaker et al., 1999).

These findings have influenced the American Academy of Pediatrics to recommend "no more than 1 to 2 hours of quality TV and videos a day for older children and no screen time for children under the age of 2" (American Academy of Pediatrics 2005). The U.S. Department of Health and Human Services (US DHHS) has established a national objective for 2010 to "increase the proportion of adolescents who view television 2 or fewer hours on a school day" (US DHHS 2000). The quantitative target for this objective is to increase this proportion of adolescents who watch 2 or fewer hours per school day to 75 percent (compared to 57 % in 1999 in the Youth Risk Behavior Surveillance System).

1.2. Study Objectives

A primary objective of this study, learning how to persuade families to adopt and adhere to the recommendation to limit children's TV viewing to 2 or fewer hours per day, is a challenge. Although parents have come to understand and express concern over the effect media use has on academic achievement as well as its social and behavioral consequences, such as aggressive behavior, parents may be less aware of the link between their child's weight and his/her media use. With the problem of childhood obesity escalating and definitive links between childhood obesity and media use by children firmly established, it is critical for researchers to begin to understand the factors that shape the amount of time children spend in front of the TV and whether the choices they make with other media contribute to or ameliorate the problems of childhood obesity.

This study explored the individual and familial forces, and parents' perceptions of community forces that shape children's television viewing with the goal of understanding the barriers and opportunities for reducing TV time to 2 hours per day or less. A diverse sample of 180 parents and their 6- to 13-year-old children participated in open-ended, small group discussions in 2003 and 2004. Participants described their typical media use patterns, their rules and strategies for limiting TV viewing, and their perspectives on the impact that reducing TV viewing would have on their children and families. In this Highlights Report, we describe points of confusion and concern expressed by parents with regard to the recommendation, along with the barriers to change that families identified. We then suggest several promising strategies to reduce TV time and media time, strategies that might ultimately reduce the risk of childhood overweight.

The study was designed to help (1) understand the forces that influence children of both sexes and of various ages and racial/ethnic backgrounds to use TV and other media involving sedentary behavior; (2) explore the challenges of and opportunities for limiting children's television viewing to 2 hours per day; and (3) develop strategies for reducing TV use that might work for families. By accomplishing these goals, we hoped to contribute to the achieving the national objective that 75 percent of adolescents will watch 2 or fewer hours of TV per school day (US DHHS 2000, Objective 22-11).

1.3. Study Methods and Approach

1.3.1. Site Selection

Data were collected between October 2003 and March 2004 in three locations: Philadelphia, PA, Chicago, IL, and Richmond, VA. These locations were chosen to capture distinct population demographics (race/ethnicity, urban/suburban area, and socioeconomic structure).

Participants in Philadelphia were recruited through elementary and middle schools and community-based organizations. Participants in Chicago and Richmond were recruited through focus group facilities (with the stipulation that families could not have participated in any other focus group during the past 12 months). Recruitment materials indicated that children and their parents would participate in a small group discussion about how children spend their out-ofschool time, particularly their television viewing habits. Families were offered an honorarium for their participation in the project. The study, its protocol, and its consent/assent forms were approved by the Institutional Review Boards of the University of Pennsylvania and RTI International (Federalwide Assurance Number 3331, project 8680).

1.3.2. Sample Selection

The study recruited pairs of a parent and his/her child (aged 6 to 7, 9 to 10, and 12 to 13) to participate in the study. In all, 180 parents and their children participated in this research. To compare differences in ages, we included children in the research if they were aged 6 to 7, 9 to 10, or 12 to 13. These groupings were chosen to reflect ages that shape children's interests and abilities, as well as their decision-making autonomy. Roughly one third of the children fell into each age category. More than three quarters of the parent participants were mothers (77 %), less than one-quarter were fathers (21.1 %), and the remainder were another caregiver, such as a grandparent. The respondents were approximately evenly divided between boys and girls. In Chicago and Richmond, the groups were constructed to be homogeneous in terms of race/ethnicity (African American, white, or Hispanic), although groups were mixed in terms of sex. The overall distribution of the sample is shown in ***Tables 1 and 2***. The socioeconomic circumstances of the families varied considerably. Although the study did not entail a random sample, the families were similar to national samples in their access to media and their patterns of media use (see Section 2.1).

1.3.3. Data Collection Procedures

Each parent/child pair came to an identified location within their community, such as the child's school, the university, or a focus group center. Each parent was asked to fill out a household media Inventory (HMI). The HMI asked about the number and location of media (i.e., television, computers, cable and Internet access, and videogame consoles) throughout the home. Parents and children also filled out background forms (BFs), which gathered socioeconomic data and information about behavior. BF questions on sedentary use of media assessed children's daily and weekly time with television, computers, and videogames; parents were asked about their child's time with the same media and about their own television use.

Table 1. Structure of Discussion Groups by Age Group.

	Chicago	Richmond	Philadelphia	Total
6 to 7 years				
Parents Children	8 groups (n = 27) 27 interviews	4 groups (n = 15) 15 interviews	6 groups (n = 19) 19 interviews	18 groups (n = 61) 61 interviews
9 to 10 years				
Parents Children	8 groups (n = 28) 8 groups (n = 28)	4 groups (n = 15) 4 groups (n = 15)	6 groups (n = 17) 6 groups (n = 17)	18 groups (n = 60) 18 groups (n = 60)
12 to 13 years				
Parents Children	8 groups (n = 25) 8 groups (n = 25)	4 groups (n = 15) 4 groups (n = 15)	8 groups (n = 19) 8 groups (n = 19)	20 groups (n = 59) 20 groups (n = 59)
Total				
Parents	24 groups (n = 80)	12 groups (n = 45)	20 groups (n = 55)	56 groups (n = 180)
Children	16 groups and 27 interviews (n = 80)	8 groups and 15 interviews (n = 45)	14 groups and 19 interviews (n = 55)	38 groups and 61 interviews (n = 180)

Table 2. Race/Ethnicity and Sex of Children by Age Group.

	Male	Female	Total
6 to 7 years			
African American	7	16	23
White (non-Hispanic)	10	10	20
Hispanic	11	5	16
Other	1	1	2
Subtotal	29	32	61
9 to 10 years			
African American	10	7	17
White (non-Hispanic)	10	13	23
Hispanic	7	9	16
Other	3	1	4
Subtotal	30	30	60
12 to 13 years			
African American	10	12	22
White (non-Hispanic)	9	12	21
Hispanic	11	4	15
Other	0	1	1
Subtotal	30	29	59
Total			
African American	27	35	62
White (non-Hispanic)	29	35	64
Hispanic	29	18	47
Other	4	3	7
Total	89	91	180

Next, parents and children engaged in separate child or adult open-ended small group interviews led by trained moderators. Discussions were held with groups of three or four parents while, in another room, discussions were conducted with groups of three or four 9- to 10-year-olds or 12- to 13-year-olds. Children aged 6 to 7 were interviewed individually. Because we learned in the pilot test that it was hard for young children to stay focused on a discussion or provide their individual responses rather than repeat each other's answers, we conducted one-on-one, open- ended interviews with the 6- to 7-year-olds. In both the children's groups and the parents' groups, participants were asked about the child's typical day, the child's media use on weekdays and weekends, rules about television and other media, the benefits and costs of television viewing, reactions to a 2-hour per day limit on TV time, and strategies for reducing TV time.

Each child also was asked to draw her or her favorite activity. Parent group discussions lasted an average of 90 minutes, children's group interviews lasted approximately 60 minutes, and one-on- one interviews lasted 30 minutes. The children were supervised by an adult in a room with play activities during the time they were not involved in the interviews.

Interviews and discussions with children were conducted in English. Hispanic parents were offered the choice of participating in a focus group discussion that was conducted in English or Spanish. Approximately one-third of the discussions with Hispanic parents were held in Spanish, and transcripts of these discussions were translated into English for analysis.

1.3.4. Data Analysis

Data from the HMIs and BFs were entered into SPSS software (version 11.5) and analyzed to provide an overview of the media use patterns of this sample and to allow for comparisons both within the sample and to media use patterns of national samples of children. Transcripts were generated from interview groups and one-on-one interviews. Whenever possible, speakers were identified by the transcriber and tagged for age, sex, race/ethnicity, and interview location (all names were replaced with ID numbers). Transcripts were thematically coded using the qualitative software program ATLAS.ti 5.0. Themes were developed on the basis of input from the investigators who moderated and observed the parents' and children's interviews.ATLAS software was used to sort quotations (demarcated by numeric IDs) by age (6 to 7, 9 to 10, 12 to 13), race (white, African American, English-speaking Hispanic, Spanish- speaking Hispanic, and other), and sex (boy, girl; mother, father). After demographic sorts were run, analysts generated MS Word documents summarizing themes and MS Excel spreadsheets summarizing numeric trends.

2. Highlights of Study Findings

2.1. Media Availability and Use

2.1.1. Media in the Home

For most children in this sample, media are ubiquitous. The HMIs reveal that the average family in this study had four working television sets in the home. Most children (64 %) had a bedroom TV, and a large proportion of the families in this sample (46 %) reported that they had a television set in an eating space such as a dining room or kitchen. The HMIs also reveal that the children in this sample lived not only in a multiple-TV environment but also in a multiple- media environment. Virtually all households (99 %) had a DVD or VCR; the vast majority had a videogame console (88 %) and a computer (85 %); and more than half had Internet access (56 %).

2.1.2. Children's Viewing Patterns

We assessed children's TV viewing from the BFs and discussions with parents and children. Parents described the children's day and the children's time with television throughout the course of an average day. Children provided this information by reporting on the television shows that they watched on the previous day. As has been reported by others (e.g., Robinson 1999), parents in this study indicated that their children watched less television than the children themselves reported (parent mean, 116 minutes; child mean, 189 minutes).

The study did not determine whether the children or the parents were more accurate reporters of the children's time with television. The children, especially younger children, had a widely varying sense of time, but they were general fairly confident in describing the specific shows they watched the prior day. In contrast, parents admitted that they found it difficult to keep track of children's time with media, and this was particularly the case with videogame use. In addition, during discussions parents asked the interviewers for clarification about what "counts" as television viewing. For example, while children may have included watching a videotaped movie with their father in their viewing estimates, the fathers may have classified that activity as time spent with their child. Moreover, several parents indicated that they considered weekdays (or school nights) and weekends (or nonschool nights) separately and that they had a better sense of some days than others

Children reported watching, on average, more than 3 hours of TV on the previous day; and only 30 percent of children watched less than 2 hours on the previous day. The amount of viewing increased by an hour or more when computers and videogames were included (see ***Figure 1***).

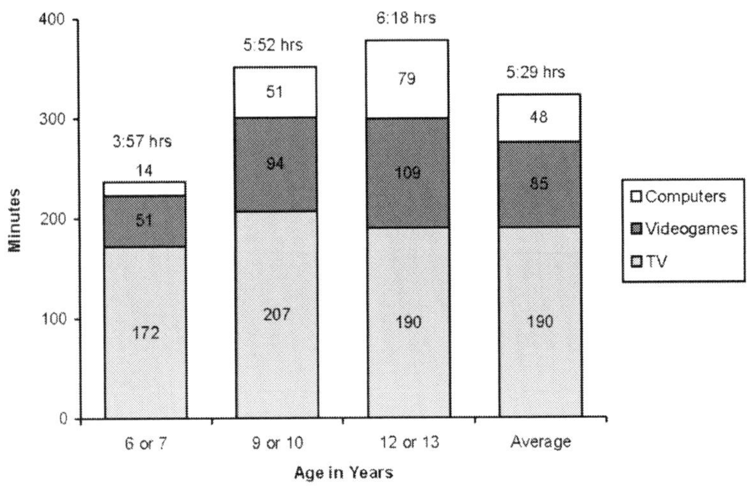

Source: RTI/APPC 2004.

Figure 1. Screen Time, by Age—Child Reports by Mean Hours and Minutes Spent "Yesterday".

Highlights of the findings on media use included the following:

- Parents in this study reported that their children watched, on average, fewer than 2 hours per day in an average week; however, children themselves reported that they watched more than 3 hours per day.
- Videogame and computer use brought children's total daily "screen time" to nearly 5 and one half hours per day—a time that parallels national data trends (APPC 2000).
- Children's reports of their media use were higher than parents' reports. The levels of the differences were similar to those observed by Robinson (1999).

2.2. Beliefs and Attitudes about Media Use

2.2.1. Children's Attitudes

The majority of the children in the study had a strong affinity to media. Even children as young as age 6 could identify their favorite TV shows, and boys expressed strong affinity for videogames.

Favorite Activities

Children were asked to provide a drawing of their favorite thing to do when they were not in school. The most striking finding was that 57 percent of the children in our study identified in-home screen media (TV, videogames, or computers) as a favorite activity (see ***Table 3***). All age groups had a similar proportion (between 54 % and 60 %) across all age groups of children. By comparison, only about a quarter (27 %) of children featured sports or physical activities in their drawings.

Among boys, the most popular activity was videogames. Videogames were featured as a favorite activity by more than half (56 %) of boys; by comparison, TV was featured by less than a quarter (22 %) of boys. Videogames appealed to boys in a variety of ways. A particular appeal of videogames is the challenge of mastering new levels:

> *A 7-year-old boy drew himself with a PS-2 hooked up to a TV screen playing Mario Party 4 because "You get to pick Mario, Luigi, or anyone you want to be on your team. If you win, you go to another game."* (7-year-old Hispanic boy)

Among girls, TV was featured more than twice as often as videogames (27 % vs. 13 %):

> *A 9-year-old girl drew a picture of herself watching a TV with the word "NICK" on the screen, while the girl said, "Yea! Nick!" and her mom came in "bringing cookies."* (9-year-old White girl)

Among girls (in contrast to boys), computers were similar in popularity to videogames (each was featured in about 13% of the drawings). Younger girls often liked the cartoon features on the computer games. Older girls featured the appeal of talking to their friends through instant messaging.

Table 3. Percent of Children whose Drawings of "Favorite Activity When Not in School" Featured Various Elements.

		Activities in the Home					Outside the Home	
		Media Activities				Nonmedia Inside Activities	Sports/ Physical Activity	General Outside
Group	N	TV	Video-games	Computer	Any Media			
Age Group								
6 to 7%	56	18	36	7	54	13	20	21
9 to 10 %	57	25	33	12	58	32	20	5
12 to 13 %	48	33	31	17	60	19	44	19
Sex								
Female %	84	27	13	13	45	30	26	19
Male %	77	22	56	12	70	12	29	10
Race/Ethnicity								
African American %	53	20	25	11	49	25	23	17
White %	57	30	37	12	58	21	40	14
Hispanic %	41	34	44	12	73	17	17	12
Total %	161	25	34	12	57	21	27	15

NOTE: If a child's drawing featured more than one activity, each of these activities was coded. Thus, for each type of activity, the percentage represents all children whose drawing included that activity. As a result, total percentages equal more than 100.

2.2.2. Parent Attitudes

Parents described both positive and negative effects of TV and other media. One mother expressed her ambivalence this way:

> *I wish she'd watch less, but my double-edged sword is if she's watching less and she has no friends, I'd become the entertainment [laughter] or the entertainer. And I just feel like I'd, you know, you juggle a whole lot during the day and of course, but the time she's bored, I'm fixing dinner. So it's still a baby-sitter at this age.* (White mother of a 12-yearold girl)

Parents reported features that they liked and disliked about TV, computers, and videogames. These likes and dislikes are shown below.

What Parents Liked

Keeping children safely occupied. About half of parents in our groups mentioned that they liked the fact that TV and media helped to keep their children safely occupied (particularly for younger children). For instance:

> *I've used it as an electronic babysitter sometimes. I need to get something done, and I know that I'll have at least a half hour if they're watching at the top of or the bottom of the hour.* (White mother of a 6-year-old boy)
>
> *Yes, unfortunately, yes, it's helpful. It helps me by keeping her busy while I'm cooking or grocery shopping. It's helpful, but perhaps we take too much advantage of it. We depend too much on that distraction, and that's wrong.* (Spanish-speaking Hispanic mother of a 9-year-old girl)
>
> *Because I work at night, so a lot of times in the day I'm asleep, so unless my husband is home or whatever, [my child] will play the Play Station or TV, and he won't be out in the street, or stuff like that.* (African American mother of a 12-year-old boy)

Media help children learn new skills or information. About a third of parents mentioned that TV provided educational benefits for children:

> *Yeah, they have a lot of stuff on cable, like, as far as history, civil rights struggle, all stuff like that. You know, they might ask questions about, "Well, this is what Martin Luther King done." So, it can be very helpful.* (African American mother of a 13-year-old boy)

Computers were often viewed favorably in terms of the educational content they may provide. Even videogames were viewed favorably in light of their positive impact on eye-hand coordination.

Media improve communication between parents and their children. About a quarter of parents mentioned that they liked watching TV together to share in a common activity or that TV provided interesting things for parents and children to talk about:

> *See, my son's the type you have to drag things out of him as far as what happened in school or, you know, what's going on. He never says anything. Now if we're watching a*

show or something and something comes up, you know, he may mention, oh, that happened, you know, the other day. So it kind of keeps me abreast of what's going on with that age group, you know. (African American mother of a 10-year-old boy)

Well, we share things with each other about the TV. And she'll come and say, "I'm going to tell you what just happened," even though it's right in the middle of something I'm watching... and we laugh. (African American mother of a 7-year-old girl)

Media help parents regulate their children's behavior. Parents mentioned that they liked the ability to use television as a reward for desired behavior, such as completing chores or homework. In addition, in some families, parents used television as a tool to help children relax and ease the transition to bedtime:

It's really a very simple way to just get them to sit down and relax because, you know, my children are very active. [My son is] very active and to me, it's nice, it's very pleasant for me when he's sort of like fed, cleaned, you know, teeth are brushed, and he's going to just sit down for a while and watch TV. It's a calm, nice thing. Now, you know, I could do other things with him at that point. (White mother of a 12-year-old boy)

What Parents Disliked

Parents also expressed concerns about the possible negative effects of TV and videogames on children. There appeared to be three sets of concerns:

Opportunity cost. Parents commonly evaluated children's media use in terms of whether the children ought to be doing something else more valuable or useful. In other words, overuse of a medium might deprive a child of more beneficial experiences and social activities, but the media themselves were not considered innately harmful:

I don't see it affecting her, but I feel like she could be doing something more productive. (English-speaking Hispanic father of a 6-year-old girl)

But also—his creativity—he does not develop it because he just sits watching television. He does not look for other ways to entertain himself like reading or doing things or going outside. (Spanish-speaking Hispanic father of a 13-year-old boy)

Since boys are, especially when they are younger, more socially challenged than girls—it hurts them or it can hurt them... You can become a hermit just by playing these games all day. (White father of a 10-year-old boy)

Psychological effects of harmful content. A minority of parents also worried that the content of TV and in particular the violence of videogames might be a bad influence on their children:

Day by day the games become more violent.
It affects their psyche.
They [videogames] are very real... the blood gushes out...
(Spanish-speaking Hispanic mothers of 9- to 10-year-old boys)

In addition, several parents objected to the commercialism of television:

One of the things that I do not like about television and one of the areas that I think affects them is consumerism. If there are some tennis shoes that are in fashion, they will see them there; if there is a shirt that is in fashion, they see it there; if there is a drink that is in... And they are the wrong messages, for example, my son now that he is wrestling says, "No, I have to drink Gatorade because they say it is better than water." Those type of things that in my opinion are harmful to them. (Spanish-speaking Hispanic father of a 12-year-old boy)

In addition to their concerns about potential consequences of media use, some parents had directly observed behaviors related to media use that they disliked:

So we had to stop them from watching, because it was really—we'd be talking to them, and they'd start talking in these funny voices, and you'll ask them something, "Can you pass me that?" and they'll make a funny noise. And I said, "See, that's it, no. You're not watching, no, because it's too much." They lose their identity in the TV. (African American mother of a 7-year-old girl)

Several parents mentioned that their children became moody or aggressive after using electronic media:

[My son] is a pill on the days that he watches TV. (White mother of a 6-year-old boy)

You know, so, um, he gets, um, zoned when he watches TV. Hypnotized. And he can't hear and he can't think, he can't do anything, so I cut it, turn off the TV. So you know it's not helpful, it's just something that he does to occupy his time. (African American mother of a 12-year-old boy)

Physical health consequences of long-term use. A few parents were concerned about the potential negative health consequences of media use on overweight.

I could just see him getting bigger watching TV, and he'd eat and go lay down and watch TV all day... I just feel that later he might gain a lot of weight by just laying down watching TV, because he'll eat and go lay down. So I tend, I really don't like him to watch it. I'd rather he did some activities or something besides that. (African American mother of a 12-year-old boy)

She would just watch it. She just sits there and eats. She'll just finish eating something and she'll get up to get something else. It's like, "You just ate a whole bag of chips. Why are you going to get more?" I mean, she just doesn't realize what she's doing and how much she's eating and how much she's watching. (White mother of a 9-year-old girl)

He does not have activities. He finishes a program and he goes to the refrigerator to look for something. And when that is over he goes to the refrigerator to see what else he can take to the living room to keep eating. And that is all day long. It affects his health. (Spanish-speaking Hispanic mother of a 12-year-old boy)

2.3. Reactions to Recommendations for Limiting TV to 2 Hours per Day

In the discussion groups, we used several approaches to elicit reactions to the recommendation that children should watch no more than 2 hours of television a day. First, we asked parents to discuss what they thought was the right amount of time for their children to spend watching TV. Next, we asked parents for their reactions to recommendations that children should watch no more than 2 hours or less (US DHHS 2000, Objective 22-11). We then asked parents and children for the reasons for limiting TV. Finally, we talked about barriers to limiting TV use.

2.3.1. Parent Perceptions of the Appropriate Amount of TV

When asked, two thirds of the parents in our study thought that the right amount of TV for their children to watch was less than 2 hours a day. Yet, while most parents said that children's television viewing on a school day should be limited to 2 hours or less, they were more generous on weekends, with the majority saying that they would allow 3 or more hours a day of viewing on weekends.

2.3.2. Reactions to the Recommendation of Limited TV

Responses to the recommendation that children watch no more than 2 hours of television a day were generally positive:

> *I think it's a good recommendation. It 's just going to be a task, you know, to enforce it, but it's worth giving it a try.* (Hispanic mother of a 9-year-old girl)
>
> *Well, it's in line with what we try to keep and maintain at home, but, I mean, I'd like to know where he came up with the 2 hours.* (White mother of a 9-year-old boy)
>
> *I do not think it would be easy... but I believe it would be better because it would give us more time for our children.* (Hispanic mother of a 10-year-old girl)

Although the majority of parents agreed in theory with 2 hours or less of TV per day, they had a number of concerns about their ability to put this into practice. They expressed concerns about their ability to get their own work done and keep their child safe and about the implication that they would have to reduce their own TV watching to avoid being hypocritical:

> *I'd like to say that I could limit [my son] to 2 hours a day. I think that would be perfect. But that would also mean that I would channel his interest in other areas and be with him throughout that time. And I can't always commit to that because of the other obligations that I have including cooking dinners, chores, and doing other things that kids require. So I think 2 hours is a perfect time. It doesn't always work.* (African American mother of a 9-year-old boy)

The majority of parents also made a distinction between their ability to adhere to the recommendation during weekdays and on the weekend, when their children's viewing was higher and the perceived need to limit it was lower. Many parents talked about how their children did not watch much during the week but watched a lot on the weekend.

Parents also asked the moderator (if he/she had not already clarified this) if the 2 hours a day included other media, such as DVDs they might rent or videogames they might play on the TV. Several parents said that they thought their child's alternative would be another electronic medium:

It depends on, does that mean videogames too? Because they'll be like [laughter], "Okay, I don't need to watch TV, Mom, just let me play." You know? (English-speaking Hispanic father of a 12-year-old boy)

2.3.3. Parent Understanding of Reasons for Limiting TV

We also asked parents what they thought were reasons that the experts might make a recommendation to limit TV viewing. Parents were most likely to say that the recommendation stems from concern over children's sedentary lifestyle and the growing problem of childhood obesity:

And I know that they're saying that they're eating more when they're sitting and sedentary, so, although mine don't, but I know that they do. (White mother of a 9-yearold girl)

I have a 25-year-old nephew who's obese because he was allowed unlimited access to the TV. (White mother of a 9-year-old girl)

Parents who listed the concern over sedentary lifestyle/childhood obesity as a reason to limit media use were not different in age or race/ethnicity from other parents. Parents of boys, however, were more likely than parents of girls to say that the recommendation is based on concern over overweight/physical inactivity.

Parents also frequently cited concern over children's cognitive development as a reason why health authorities might recommend limits on TV viewing. Interestingly, while parents of boys were more likely to list concern over the sedentary nature of TV viewing, parents of girls were more likely to list concern over how it might affect their daughter's school performance. Parents of 9- to 10-year-olds were the most likely to talk about TV and school performance, and, as the following quote below illustrates, the concern was not limited to parents of girls. This woman, in addition to describing concern over her son's weight, echoed the sentiment of other parents of 9- to 10-year-olds:

I mean, yeah, the education part of it because, well, I mean, when they're younger, I mean, I'm not saying their schoolwork was easier but they had better grade averages before. And now [my son's] below average, so I think... It has an effect on him and I think it comes from the parent too, you know, if I go to work and I come home and use the excuse that I'm too tired or whatever and I don't take more time out with him. So I think if I monitor that television watching or videogame playing and spend more time doing that then it would help. (English-speaking Hispanic mother of a 9-year-old boy)

The third most commonly cited belief about the reasoning behind the recommendation was concern over content. This issue was more often discussed by African American parents, parents of older children, and parents of boys. These parents described mainly the deleterious effects of viewing sex and violence:

That's how kids today, you know, they're learning how to do so much evil, you know, because there's a whole lot of evil on TV, too, you know, and everything people make, you know, has got killing in it, you know, or you got sex in it, you know? So I think that that might be the reason why he said 2-hour limit, you know? ... So that they won't hey, just sit there and that's the only thing that turns them on is what's on TV, you know? (African American mother of a 12-year-old girl)

2.3.4. Children's Perceptions of Reasons for Limiting TV

We also asked children what they thought about a 2-hour limit on TV time and what they thought were the reasons that parents might want to limit the amount of TV they watched. As might be expected, more children than parents said that 2 hours a day was too little. The 9- to 10- year-olds tended to be more fervent in arguing against it:

> *I'd go insane.* [Moderator: "So what would you ...?"] *Put up a big protest.* (9-year-old white boy)

Boys were primarily concerned about the effects of limiting TV on their videogame playing:

> *When you say that, do you include like watching TV and videogames too? 'Cause most videogames you gotta hook up to the TV.* (9- to 10-year-old mixed-race boy)

The 6- to 7-year-old children were more compliant:

> *I've been on a train with my mother, and I told her, "Mommy, I'll do anything for you."* (6-year-old Hispanic girl)

It was interesting that even 6- to 7-year-old children could articulate the reasons for limiting TV. The most salient to the children was the impact of television on their cognitive development. They talked about the potential effect of TV on their brains, on their homework, and on their school performance:

> *Because she wants me to learn, learn the hard way, not just by watching TV. Not that she's being mean, but she wants me to learn by hard work and concentration.* (6-year-old mixed-race boy)
>
> *Because I think they believe the thing is, you watch too much TV, your brain turns into mush—your brain turns to mush, and then we have to spend money getting you a new brain.* (9-year-old African American boy)

Children could also cite reasons associated with their behavior. One group of 9- to 10-year-old children listed the following reasons why parents might want to limit the amount of time children spend watching TV; these comments reflect the reasons given by many children:

> *They get dumb.*
> *They get in trouble with school.*
> *They don't get fun to play with.*
> *They start swearing too much.*

2.4. Current Rules for Limiting Media Use

Parents and children were asked what rules or practices they had about TV use. Responses were analyzed by age, sex, and ethnicity. In general, both parents and children were specifically asked if they had any rules about media time or content, but parents were much more descriptive and tended to spontaneously elaborate on their media practices. Hence, much of the analysis here focuses on the perceptions of parents.

Nearly all the parents in our groups reported practices or rules to restrict their children's television viewing. These practices fall under four broad categories: content restriction or monitoring, activity or behavior contingency, duration, and availability.

2.4.1. Rules about Content

Most parents in our study reported rules that restricted the content of TV that they would allow their children. Parents were often concerned about exposure to sexual content, violence, or foul language.

The nature of these rules ranged from limiting access to specific shows or channels, to allowing only certain types of programs (namely, educational), to allowing "no talk shows" or only shows that depicted characters of the same age as the child. Other rules included not allowing a child to touch the remote control and requiring the child to ask permission before watching a particular show. A small number of parents (less than 10 %) controlled content with practices that limited access to TV, such as not putting a TV in a child's bedroom, not installing cable TV, or using a V-chip to limit the channels a child could watch.

Even young children could explain the practices their families had about content. Interviews with African American 6- to 7-year-olds produced reports of the following practices:

No grown-up shows.
No nasty talk.
No swearing on it.

2.4.2. Rules regarding Homework and Chores

About half the parents reported that they allowed TV only if certain activities were completed. About a third of these parents reported that their child must finish homework before watching television. Parents generally had the attitude that as long as their children's homework was complete, they could and should be allowed to watch TV or play with other media. A handful said that their children could watch television provided that all their chores, such as cleaning their room and doing their homework, were complete. Children generally accepted these practices or rules as a part of their daily routine.

2.4.3. Practices Limiting the Duration of TV Viewing

Almost half of parents described rules limiting media time, but at least half of these appeared to be understood family practices rather than clearly articulated rules such as only 2 hours of TV. These family practices were often dependent on a parent's sense that his or her child had watched too much television.

Behavioral Monitoring

About a quarter of parents reported that they knew when their child had watched too much TV and it was time to shut the TV off:

> *I guess when you, you know, you look at the clock and you're like, "Gosh, it's been an hour and they've been sitting there the whole hour. Isn't there anything else, you know, that they could...," you know, I'll say, "Is your room clean? Are your chores done?" And then if everything's, "Yeah, yeah, yeah," then its like, "Okay, well, that's enough." You know, there's, you know, "The TV's been on long enough." I guess I mean, for me after an hour it's like, if I'm in the kitchen and I can hear it, you know, it just gets on my nerves. [Laughter] I'm like, "Okay, that's enough, you know, go outside, get out and do something."* (White mother of a 13-year-old boy)

Some parents said they allowed their child to watch some TV and after a certain time or number of shows, parents would tell the children to take a break and engage in another activity. The reasoning behind this strategy stems from the parents' desire to prevent kids from zoning out before it's too late, to distract the child with another activity, and reduce the child's desire to watch more television—in other words, to prevent TV from becoming a default activity:

> *It's not like any concrete rules, um, if he's not listening or in tune to what I'm saying, the TV goes off, 'cause I see he's in a zone with the TV, and then he'll, um, he'll come back to earth (laughter), and he'll do what he's supposed to do.* (African American mother of a 13-year-old boy)
>
> *She gets very unhappy if I turn it off after a period of time and she doesn't know what to do with herself. I call that TV brain. So I stop it after a certain period of time when I notice that she's zoning out.* (White mother of a 12-year-old girl)

Clear Rules about the Duration of TV Viewing

Only about a quarter of families reported clear rules about the duration of TV viewing. The most common practice with younger children involved not allowing TV viewing past a certain time of day. Among parents of 9- to 10-year-old children, the most common practice was not allowing TV viewing during weekdays. Among the parents of 12- to 13-year-olds, the most common practice to limit TV use was to establish a specific amount of allowable TV use. In most instances where rules existed about the duration of TV viewing, the limits were less than 2 hours. However, only a minority of families had these types of rules.

Clear practices to limit the duration of TV viewing are slightly more common among younger children than older children and among white and Hispanic parents than among African American parents. There were no appreciable differences by sex.

Another challenge is that rules about the duration of TV viewing were generally relaxed on weekends. And many parents think that their children have a right to relax on the weekend.

> *It would not be good to set a time ...I believe the weekend is for them to do as they please.* (Spanish-speaking Hispanic mother of 6- to 7-year-old boy)
>
> *Go ahead. Do your thing. You wanna sit with the computer, play games, and watch TV all day that's all right, so long as you spend the other 4 days, the other 5 days without it.* (African American parent of 9- to 10-year-old girl)

2.5. Barriers to Reducing TV Time

The next portion of our discussion explored barriers to reducing children's TV time. It was apparent that in order to get children to watch less TV, parents need to support this reduction. This study identified a number of barriers to limiting TV use by parents.

2.5.1. Failure to Recognize a Problem

In general, the parents did not have a problem with the amount of TV their child watched. They commented that they would become concerned if their child started having problems in school or had behavioral problems. Parents noted:

> *As long as he's doing OK in school and he can keep up his grades, he can keep his TV.* (Hispanic mother of a 12-year-old boy)
>
> *They've always done homework in front of the TV or with the stereos on, and they get good grades so how can I tell them it's not good if they're getting As and Bs?* (Mother of a 9-year-old)
>
> *But if a note arrives from school that he misbehaved or whatever, then he is punished the next day... The next day he does not watch television.* (Spanish-speaking Hispanic mother of a 7-year-old boy)
>
> *As long as he handles his responsibilities and gets done what he needs to get done, everything is okay.* (Mother of a 9-year-old boy)

While parents recognized, in principle, the relationship between TV and overweight, they did not see the risk as applying to their own children. For instance, one mother said:

> *A lot of kids are overweight for they are couch potatoes. I feel bad for them, because they've got weight they can't take off. But not my kids.* (Hispanic mother of a 12-year-old boy)

2.5.2. Reliance on TV as a Babysitter and Concern about Becoming an Entertainer

Parents also indicated reluctance to give up the use of TV as a babysitter to keep their children entertained as the parents did housework, cooked, or found time for themselves. For instance, several mothers commented:

> *Oh, it's just a phenomenal babysitter. If everybody in the house needs to be doing things, it's just fabulous.* (White mother of a 9-year-old girl)
>
> *No TV? How would I cook?* (African American mother of a 7-year-old girl)

Other parents expressed concerns about needing to become an entertainer if they limited TV.

> *I can't entertain him all day.* (African American mother of a 9-year-old boy)
>
> *If she watches less, I become the entertainer. And I'm cooking dinner.* (White mother of a 12-year-old girl)

Ironically, parents may perceive a bigger barrier in this area than may actually be the case. When parents were asked what they would do as an alternative to TV, parents described themselves as needing to be actively involved with their children, while the children typically described alternative activities in which they entertained themselves.

2.5.3. Hassle and Conflict

Other parents expressed concern that limiting TV would create additional hassles in their home; this was more often the case when there were several children. For instance, one mother explained:

> *I would give them the cartoons to stop the commotion. I would prefer to see them play, but sometimes I just want to sit and look* [at TV]. (African American mother of a 7-yearold boy)

2.5.4. Reluctance to Reduce Their Own TV Use

Parents who enjoyed watching television themselves realized that to cut down on their children's TV time, they would need to reduce their own use. Often they were reluctant to make that change. One mother said:

> *Well, I think my husband and I would really have to get out of the comfort zone of sitting down and watching TV as well.* (Hispanic mother of a 12-year-old girl)

More detail about barriers to changing TV use is provided in the next section, where we discuss specific changes that a family might make.

2.6. Reactions and Barriers to Potential Changes

To more thoroughly explore the barriers and possible incentives to changes, we asked parents to discuss four specific strategies that, if implemented, would have the result of reducing children's TV use. By doing this, we sought to understand family reactions to more incremental change strategies. We explored (1) no background TV, (2) no TV during mealtimes, (3) no TV in children's bedrooms, and (4) no afternoon TV. We selected the afternoon because it seemed to be the time of day during which TV viewing is most prevalent.

2.6.1. Parent Reactions to Suggestions for No Background TV

In general, parents seemed agreeable to the strategy of removing background TV. Most agreed that it was a good strategy and that it would be easy to implement. Of the four suggested strategies, this was the one that parents generally felt would be easiest to implement. Some even mentioned that they had already tried to reduce background TV in their homes by turning off the TV when no one was watching.

Yet, even parents who agreed that it was a good idea to turn off background TV noted that enforcement of this rule would require them to be more active in turning off the TV. Moreover, a minority of parents (nearly a quarter of the parents who made comments about this suggested change) were resistant to this strategy, suggesting that they were the "culprits" because they liked the background noise themselves. Interestingly, there seemed to be some guilt associated with the responses from these parents. It may be that they realized that, although it would be good for their child, it would be an unlikely strategy for them to implement:

> *I think I leave the television on to avoid the noise with [my daughter] and my younger son because they are always really loud and I can't take a lot of noise.* (African American mother of a 7-year-old girl)
>
> *I like having the background noise. Could we do it? Sure [laughter], I would probably be the one to object more so than anybody else.* (White mother of a 12-year-old girl)

2.6.2. Parent Reactions to No Mealtime TV

For many parents, no TV during mealtime seemed to be a good strategy. Some parents mentioned that watching TV while eating meals did not occur in their household. Interestingly, however, a lot of these parents were quick to distinguish snacks from meals, noting that they did eat snacks while watching TV. Some parents also mentioned that occasionally they ate pizza while watching TV and perceived this activity as a treat for the whole family.

On the other hand, a minority of parents (perhaps 10 % of the total sample, but 30 % of respondents who currently had TV on during mealtime), had negative reactions to this suggestion. Of the parents who commented that they had the TV on during mealtime, nearly twice as many expressed a favorable reaction to the change as those who expressed a negative reaction. Negative reactions to eliminating TV during mealtime were nearly twice as common among parents of 6- to 7-year-olds than among parents of older children.

The barriers to change among these parents stemmed from the perceived benefits that derived from the TV's ability to distract children, resulting in less bickering among family members during mealtimes. Some parents reported that mealtimes were a time in which the family could watch the news together, allowing children to learn and ask questions about current events, and that watching TV is a stimulating and enjoyable activity:

> *It's possible, but it's stimulating for us to eat and see the events—what's going on—like the news or Jeopardy.* (Mother of a 9-year-old boy)
>
> *It's a great idea, but the bickering and everyone wants to talk, and I just need that distraction.* (Mother of a 7-year-old)

2.6.3. Parent Reactions to No TV in Children's Bedroom

In principle, parents agreed that the strategy of not having a TV in a child's bedroom would be a good way to reduce the overall amount of TV viewing. At the same time, however, many parents did not think it was an appropriate or necessary strategy for their own child. Only a third of the children in the sample did not have a TV in their bedroom. Removing a TV from a child's bedroom was perceived as particularly difficult. Indeed, there were as many negative responses to the idea of no TV in a child's bedroom as there were positive ones. Many of the negative responses dealt with the difficulty of removing a TV—one mother described this as "World War III." But parents were also concerned about the behavior that may have prompted them to put a TV in a child's bedroom in the first place. One mother commented:

No TV in my kid's bedrooms. That would be punishing me. They would never agree on what to watch. They would forever be bickering. (White mother of a 10-year-old boy)

The parents' perception was that it would be easier not to put a TV in a bedroom than to take it out. For instance, one mother explained:

Thankfully she doesn't have a [TV with a videogame] system in her room as she would be completely glued to it. You could drive a car in the room and she wouldn't notice. (White mother of a 13-year-old girl)

2.6.4. Parent Reactions to No Afternoon TV

Many parents seemed to agree with the strategy of having no afternoon TV, and many said that their child did not watch a lot of TV in the afternoon anyway. The primary reason cited by most parents was that children were doing homework then. It was common for parents to state that, after school, their child had to do homework before watching any TV. Some parents viewed TV watching as a reward for the child after homework was done.

On the other hand, roughly as many parents were resistant to the idea of no afternoon TV as were positive about the idea. A primary reason for their reluctance was that parents viewed the afternoon as a time for the child to unwind after getting home from school or a means by which the child remained occupied while parents completed household chores (e.g., cooking). For instance, mothers of 9- to 10-year-old boys said:

I think TV is fine. They need to unwind too.
That's my son's release. Because he tries so hard in school.

A few mentioned it would be a difficult strategy for them to implement because they worked and were not home with their child during the afternoon or because they would be pressed to find alternative activities for their child.

2.7. Incentives for Change

In exploring incentives for change, we asked parents and children to describe how they would feel or react to reducing TV time and what other activities they would turn to in that case. In general, children reported that they would find other ways to occupy their time.

Parents were often quite positive about the potential impact on their families of reducing TV time, citing closer family communication as the primary benefit. They were often particularly concerned about the effects of separate TV viewing in children's rooms.

Watching TV together gives you more family life.. . because, if not, each one is in their own world. (Hispanic mother of a 6-year-old girl

My sister said, "Don't you think it is not good that you have so many TVs?" That only divides the family. (Hispanic mother of a 12-year-old boy)

Some parents mentioned improved school performance as a benefit to limiting TV.

I want children to be smarter, to be able to solve problems, to be able to interact with others. If you are always in front of the TV, then the less you are getting with a real person. (White father of a 7-year-old boy)

Parents also observed behavioral improvements when their children watched less TV.

I limit the amount of TV after 6:00 pm and I notice that he is calmer without TV. (Hispanic mother of a 6-year-old boy)

My son is much more friendly and open. (White mother of a 6-year-old boy)

Nonetheless, parents were also cognizant of the potential for conflict and discontent that would ensue, not only between the child and parent but between siblings who would be spending more time interacting without TV to distract them. Hence, while parents were often aware of the positive benefits of less TV viewing, they were concerned about the consequences involved in "making it happen." Parents were apprehensive that limiting TV time would require them to be more involved in finding alternative activities for their children.

Interestingly, while most children reported that they could fairly readily find things to do on their own, parents believed they would need to be much more involved in the process by either enrolling them in classes, taking them places, spending "quality time" with them, or directly supervising children's adherence to the TV limits. However, the variety of alternatives that most children readily turned to did not involve parental involvement. This finding suggests that parents may not need to play the role of "social director" to implement a 2-hour limit. Thus, the task of reducing TV time may not be as onerous as some parents perceived.

3. Summary and Discussion of Possible Strategies

3.1. Summary

This study points to a number of challenges in effectively communicating with families about limiting children's media use. Media is deeply embedded in the life of the family, and one implication of this study is that information, by itself, may not be sufficient to move families to change their behavior. Parents generally agree with a 2-hour limit to children's TV use. It is consistent with their own views, and they understand the reasons for the recommendation, including improved education performance, positive behavior changes, and, less prominently, avoidance of obesity. Children's reactions to the idea of limiting media use are similar to those of their parents. Nevertheless, they would not like turning off media and would try to wheedle out of the limits. Thus, monitoring is important, although children indicated that they would comply with their parents' rules, as long as parents were consistent.

It is also useful to remember that families have rules about media use, particularly about content and about homework/chores. Their children tell us that they obey the rules that are enforced. Moreover, when rules about duration exist, the rules require fewer than 2 hours of use.

This study also indicated that less than a quarter of families have clear rules about duration (and even these rules are relaxed on weekends or at times when a child is watching with their parent). Moreover, media use by children in the home is pervasive. Media use data show that two thirds of children have a TV in their bedroom, and one-half of families have a TV in an eating area. As a result, children in this study are watching, on average, between 3 and 3.5 hours of TV a day and their total media use, including computers and videogames, is between 4 and 6 hours a day.

Families also report a number of barriers to limiting media use. For example, many do not perceive media use as a problem for their family. Also, parents are reluctant to change their own TV viewing, and they often rely on TV as a babysitter and to avoid conflicts and arguments. Parents are also concerned about having to become an entertainer if they cannot use TV to keep their children occupied.

Nonetheless, the study also identified possible incentives that parents expressed for reducing media use. These include increased closeness as a family, improved educational performance, improved health, and improved behavior.

The challenge is to build on this understanding, to build on current family practices for media use, and to support family values by suggesting incentives that will help to overcome the barriers to change. Because information alone is not sufficient to result in change, we must learn how to move parents to action. One model of health behavior – the Transtheoretical or "Stages of Change" model of Prochaska and DiClemente (1983; 1991) refers to the challenge of moving from "precontemplation" to "contemplation" and "preparation for action." To accomplish this, it may be useful to offer cogent reasons for reducing children's media use and to suggest actions that parents can take to make it easier to limit their children's media use.

3.2. Issues to Consider in Developing Messages for Families about Media

The findings of the study, described above, led us to identify the following as issues that are important to address in developing messages about TV viewing for families.

3.2.1. Consider Providing Broader, More Compelling Messages about Negative Effects of Excessive TV Viewing

Consideration should be given to whether parents would be more persuaded by a single focused argument, such as the connection between TV viewing and the risk of overweight, or by the accumulation of evidence about TV viewing in a variety of domains. Many parents did make the TV viewing/childhood obesity connection, but only after they were "primed" (that is, when we told them about recommendation for TV limits). Prior to this point in the discussion, their concerns about the negative effects of TV were centered on how it affected children's cognitive development (their brain, their schoolwork) and their behavior ("zombie," aggressive), but only rarely did they talk about obesity or physical inactivity. In addition, parents wanted a good rationale to present to their children for making any changes.

3.2.2. Define the 2-Hour Limit

Parents want clarity about the meaning of the recommendation to limit children's TV use. They would ask, "Does this mean 2 hours a day *every day* or 2 hours a day *averaged over the course of a week*?" Some parents do have rules restricting TV time, but the rules are considerably loosened on weekends. When asked to report how much time children spend watching TV in an average week, the mean time for average daily viewing was fewer than 2 hours a day (mean = 116 minutes). Moreover, although the majority of parents said they saw the 2-hour recommendation as reasonable, many felt that it would not work on the weekends, particularly during the winter. (There is some evidence in the literature that children's heavy viewing during the school year is more predictive of obesity than their heavy viewing during the summer [Armstrong et al. 1998].)

3.2.3. Recognize Families' Widely Differing Rules and Practices

Parents and children reported that television viewing was used as an incentive and a reward, while television restriction was used as a punishment. In addition, while some parents had very clear and consistent rules about television (e.g., limited viewing on weekdays), others had no rules about time at all. Thus, one must consider whether it is useful to construct a message about "moving the needle" (i.e., making incremental progress toward a desired objective). Would this approach have the advantage of offering something that is realistic for all families? Or would it have the danger of conveying complacency among families who do not consider their children's viewing to be a problem?

3.2.4. Build on the Incentives of Parenting

Parents feel positive and somewhat wistful about the time they spend with their children. Perhaps the most memorable portion of the discussion with parents and children was about quality time together. Several parents described their practice of scheduling "family time." It is important to recognize that television plays some role in bringing families together, and that co- viewing may not be considered in parents' calculations of the time their children spent watching TV. Strategies or messages to reduce TV time could appeal to parents' wish to spend more quality time with their children and could suggest practical ways to accomplish this without television.

3.2.5. Tailor Messages to Specific Audiences

The data suggest that there may be important ethnic, sex, and age-group differences to consider. For example, although ethnicity is conflated with interview locale variables, it appears that the Hispanic children in our sample were especially fond of videogames and that the Hispanic parents were particularly motivated by the idea of increased family communications that might result from decreased TV consumption. Moreover, girls showed different media use preferences and patterns than did boys. Girls were more resistant to TV time limits, in part because they had fewer appealing media alternatives (such as videogames). Most clear were age differences in media use and parental concerns. Parents of 9- to 10-year-olds saw time spent with computers as particularly valuable, but parents of 12- to 13-year-olds expressed concern over the perils of the Internet.

REFERENCES

[1] American Academy of Pediatrics. (2005). *Media Guidelines for Parents*. Available at: www.aap.org

[2] Anderson, R. E., Crespo, C. J., Bartlett, S. J., Cheskin, L. J. & Pratt, M. (1998). Relationship of physical activity and television watching with body weight and level of fatness among children. Results from the 3rd NHANES. *Journal of the American Medical Association, 279*, 93 8–942.

[3] Annenberg Public Policy Center. (2000). *Media in the Home: The Fifth Annual Survey of Parents and Children*. University of Pennsylvania: Philadelphia.

[4] Armstrong, C. A., Sallis, J. F., Alcaraz, J. E., Kolody, B., McKenzie, T. L. & Howell, M. F. (1998). Children's television viewing, body fat, and physical fitness. *American Journal of Health Promotion, 112*, 363–368.

[5] Center on Media and Child Health. (2005). *The Effects of Electronic Media on Children Ages Zero to Six: A History of Research*. Issue brief prepared for Kaiser Family Foundation. Boston: Center on Media and Child Health, Children's Hospital Boston.

[6] Crespo, C. J., Smit, E., Troiano, R. P., Bartlett, S. J., Macera, C. A. & Anderson, R. E. (2001). Television watching, energy intake and obesity in US children: results from the 3rd NHANES: 1988–1994. *Archives of Pediatric and Adolescent Medicine, 155*, 360–365.

[7] DiClemente, C. C., Prochaska, O., Fairhurst, S. K., Velcer, W. F., Velasquez, M. M. & Rossi, J. S. (1991). The process of smoking cessation: an analysis of precontemplation, contemplation, and preparation stages of change. *Journal of Consulting and Clinical Psychology, 59(2)*, 295–304.

[8] Dietz, W. H. & Gortmaker, S. L. (1985). Do we fatten our children at the television set? *Pediatrics, 75*, 807–812.

[9] Gorley, T., Marshall, S. J. & Biddle, S. J. H. (2004). Couch kids: correlates of television viewing among youth. *International Journal of Behavioral Medicine, 11(3)*, 152–163.

[10] Gortmaker, S. L., Must, A., Sobol, A. M., Peterson, K., Colditz, G. A. & Dietz, W. H. (1996). Television viewing as a cause of increasing obesity among children in the U.S., 1986–1990. *Archives of Pediatric and Adolescent Medicine, 150*, 356–362.

[11] Gortmaker, S. L., Peterson, K., Wiecha, J. L., Sobol, A. M., Dixit, S. & Fox, M. K., et al. (1999). Reducing obesity via a school-based interdisciplinary intervention among youth: Planet Health. *Archives of Pediatric and Adolescent Medicine, 153*, 409–418.

[12] Hedley, A. A., Ogden, C. L., Johnson, C. L., Carroll, M. D., Curtin, L. R. & Flegal, K. M. (2004). Overweight and obesity among US children, adolescents, and adults, 1999–2002. *Journal of the American Medical Association, 291*, 2847–2850.

[13] Institute of Medicine. 2005. *Preventing Childhood Obesity: Health in the Balance*. Washington, DC: National Academies Press.

[14] Lowery, S. A. & Defleur, M. L. (1995). The Iowa study of hybrid seed corn. In: (Lowery, SA, ed.).

[15] Milestones in Mass Communication Research: Media Effects. White Plains, NY: *Longman*, 115-134.

[16] Mossberg, H. O. (1989). 40-year follow-up of overweight children. *Lancet, 2*, 491–493.

[17] Prochaska, J. O. & DiClemente, C. C. (1983). *The Transtheoretical Approach.* Homewood, IL: Dow Jones Irving.

[18] Roberts, D. F., Foehr, U. G. & Rideout, V. (2005). Generation M: Media in the Lives of8–1 8 Year Olds. Palo Alto, CA: Kaiser Family Foundation.

[19] Roberts, D. F., Foehr, U. G., Rideout, V. J. & Brodie, M. (1999). *Kids & Media @ the New Millennium.* Menlo Park, CA: The Henry J. Kaiser Family Foundation.

[20] Robinson, T. N. (1999). Reducing children's television viewing to prevent obesity: a randomized controlled trial. *Journal of the American Medical Association, 282*, 1561–1567.

[21] Robinson, T. N., Killen, J. D., Kraemer, H. C., Wilson, D. M., Matheson, D. M., Haskell, W. L., et al. (2003). Dance and reducing television viewing to prevent weight gain in African American girls: the Stanford GEMS Pilot Study. *Ethnicity and Disease* 13:rfS1–65(S1–77).

[22] Signorelli, N. & Staples, J. (1997). Television and children's conceptions of nutrition. *Health Communication, 9*, 289–301.

[23] Strauss, R. S. & Pollack, H. A. (2001). Epidemic increase in childhood overweight, 1986–1998. *Journal of the American Medical Association, 286*, 2845–2848.

[24] U.S. Department of Health and Human Services. (2000). *Healthy People 2010.* 2nd edition. With Understanding and Improving Health and Objectives for Improving Health. 2 vols. Washington, DC: U.S. Government Printing Office.

[25] Woodard, E. H. & Gridina, N. (2000). *Media in the Home: The Fourth Annual Survey of Parents and Children.* Philadelphia: Annenberg Public Policy Research Center.

CHAPTER SOURCES

Chapter 1 - This is an edited, reformatted and augmented version of a White House Task Force publication, Report to the President on Childhood Obesity, dated May, 2010.

Chapter 2 - This is an edited, reformatted and augmented version of a Congressional Research Service publication, R41420, dated September 21, 2010.

Chapter 3 - This is an edited, reformatted and augmented version of a U.S. Department of Health and Human Services publication, Office of the Surgeon General, dated January, 2010.

Chapter 4 - This is an edited, reformatted and augmented version of a U.S. Department of Health and Human Services publication, Morbidity and Mortality Weekly Report, Vol.58/No.28, dated July 24, 2009.

Chapter 5 - This is an edited, reformatted and augmented version of a Research Triangle Institute publication, prepared for the Centers for Disease control and Prevention, dated March, 2007.

INDEX

A

B

D

G

H

M

N

O

P

T